D1525037

Hormone Use and Abuse by Athletes

Endocrine Updates

Series editor: Shlomo Melmed

For other titles published in this series, go to
www.springer.com/series/5917

Ezio Ghigo • Fabio Lanfranco
• Christian J. Strasburger
Editors

Hormone Use and Abuse
by Athletes

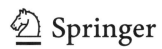 Springer

Editors
Ezio Ghigo
University of Torino
Division of Endocrinology
and Diabetology Metabolism
Department of Internal Medicine
Torino, Italy
ezio.ghigo@unito.it

Christian J. Strasburger
Charité-Universitätsmedizin
Division of Clinical Endocrinology
Department of Medicine
Campus Mitte
Berlin, Germany
Christian.Strasburger@charite.de

Fabio Lanfranco
University of Torino
Division of Endocrinology
and Diabetology Metabolism
Department of Internal Medicine
Torino, Italy
fabio.lanfranco@unito.it

ISBN 978-1-4419-7013-8   e-ISBN 978-1-4419-7014-5
DOI 10.1007/978-1-4419-7014-5
Springer New York Dordrecht Heidelberg London

Printed on acid-free paper

Springer is part of Springer Science+Business Media (www.springer.com)

Preface

Physical activity exerts an important influence on the endocrine system, modulating synthesis and secretion of several hormones. Almost every organ and system in the body is affected by physical activity and exercise, mainly through the endocrine and neuroendocrine system. Mode, intensity, and duration of the exercise bout, age, gender, and fitness level of the individual as well as environmental and psychological factors may affect the endocrine response to physical activity.

On the other hand, several hormones are able to influence physical performance and body composition. Thus, a biunivocal interrelationship between exercise and hormones exists.

In this book, new developments on metabolic and endocrine response to exercise are revised and the "hot topic" of hormonal doping in sports is introduced. In the past decades, hormone abuse has become a widespread habit among professional and – most of all and more frequently – recreational athletes. A substantial part of this volume is devoted to the effects of exogenous hormones on performance. Anabolic steroids, growth hormone and erythropoietin properties, use and misuse in sports are widely described. Specific methods to detect hormone abuse are presented and discussed.

The contributors to this volume are well-known experts and dedicated researchers in the fields of sports medicine and endocrinology, endocrine physiology, pharmacology, and doping detection.

The purpose of this volume is to provide all professionals involved in sports medicine and endocrinology a state-of-the-art overview of the complex interactions between physical activity and the endocrine system and to focus on hormone abuse in sports at competitive and recreational level highlighting its negative consequences for long-term health.

Contents

Contributors

Shehzad Basaria
Boston Claude D. Pepper Older Americans Independence Center for Function
Promoting Therapies, Section of Endocrinology, Diabetes, and Nutrition,
Boston University School of Medicine, Boston MA 02118, USA

Andrea Benso
Division of Endocrinology, Diabetology and Metabolism,
Department of Internal Medicine, University of Torino, Torino, Italy

Ignacio Bernabeu
Department of Medicine, Santiago de Compostela University, Complejo
Hospitalario Universitario de Santiago, CIBER de Fisiopatología Obesidad y
Nutrición, Instituto Salud Carlos III, Santiago de Compostela, Spain

Shalender Bhasin
Boston Claude D. Pepper Older Americans Independence Center for Function
Promoting Therapies, Section of Endocrinology, Diabetes, and Nutrition, Boston
University School of Medicine, Boston, MA 02118, USA

Martin Bidlingmaier
Endocrine Laboratory, Medizinische Klinik – Innenstadt, Ludwig-Maximilians-
University, Munich, Germany

Felipe Casanueva
Professor of Medicine, Head of the Service of Endocrinology, Clinical Hospital
of Santiago, Department of Medicine, Santiago de Compostela University, CIBER
de Fisiopatologia Obesidad y Nuricion, Santiago De Compostela, Spain

Luca Chiovato
Chair of Endocrinology Fondazione Salvatore Maugeri Istituto di Ricovero e
Cura a Carattere Scientifico, University of Pavia, Pavia, Italy

Karen Choong
Section of Endocrinology, Diabetes, and Nutrition,
Boston University School of Medicine, Boston MA, USA

Pierpaolo de Feo
Department of Internal Medicine, C.U.R.I.A.MO (Centro Universitario Ricerca
Interdipartimentale Attività Motoria), University of Perugia, Perugia, Italy

Martin Duclos
Professor Department of Sport Medicine, University of Clermont,
Clermont-Ferrand, France

Eva Fernandez
Department of Medicine, Santiago de Compostela University, Complejo
Hospitalario Universitario de Santiago, CIBER de Fisiopatología Obesidad y
Nutrición, Instituto Salud Carlos III, Santiago de Compostela, Spain

Ulrich Flenker
German Sport University Cologne, Manfred Donike Institute,
Cologne, Germany

Enrico Gabellieri
Fondazione Salvatore Maugeri Istituto di Ricovero e Cura a Carattere Scientifico,
Chair of Endocrinology, University of Pavia, Via S. Maugeri 10, 21700 Pavia, Italy

Ezio Ghigo
Professor Division of Endocrinology, Diabetology and Metabolism,
Department of Internal Medicine, University of Torino, Torino, Italy

Anthony C. Hackney
Applied Physiology Laboratory, Department of Exercise & Sport Science,
Department of Nutrition – School of Public Health, University of North Carolina,
Fetzer Building – CB # 8700, Chapel Hill, NC 27599-8700, USA

Ken K.Y. Ho
Pituitary Research Unit, Department of Endocrinology, Garvan Institute of
Medical Research (AN, KH), St. Vincent's Hospital (KH), Sydney,
NSW 2010, Australia

Ravi Jasuja
Section of Endocrinology, Diabetes, and Nutrition,
Boston University School of Medicine, Boston MA, USA

Wolfgang Jelkmann
Institute of Physiology, University of Luebeck, Ratzeburger Allee 160,
D-23538 Luebeck, Germany

Séverine Lamon
Laboratoire Suisse d'Analyse du Dopage, Centre Hospitalier Universitaire
Vaudois, University of Lausanne, Epalinges, Switzerland

Fabio Lanfranco
Division of Endocrinology, Diabetology and Metabolism,
Department of Internal Medicine, University of Torino, Torino, Italy

Anne B. Loucks
Department of Biological Sciences, Ohio University, Athens, OH, USA

Monica Marazuela
Endocrinology Section, Hospital de la Princesa, Madrid, Spain

Marco Alessandro Minetto
Division of Endocrinology and Metabolism, Department of Internal Medicine,
University of Turin, Turin, Italy

Anne E. Nelson
Pituitary Research Unit, Department of Endocrinology, St. Vincent's Hospital,
Garvan Institute of Medical Research, Sydney, Australia

Maria Kristina Parr
Institute of Biochemistry, German Sport University Cologne, Cologne, Germany

Neil Robinson
Centre Hospitalier Universitaire Vaudois, Laboratoire Suisse d'Analyse du
Dopage, University of Lausanne, Epalinges, Switzerland

Alan D. Rogol
Riley Hospital for Children, Indiana University School of Medicine,
Indianapolis, IN, USA
and
University of Virginia, Charlottesville, VA, USA

Martial Saugy
Laboratoire Suisse d'Analyse du Dopage, Centre Universitaire Romand de
Médecine Légale, Centre Hospitalier Universitaire Vaudois and University
of Lausanne, Epalinges, Switzerland

Wilhelm Schänzer
Professor German Sport University Cologne, Institute of Biochemistry,
Cologne, Germany

Jordi Segura
Bioanalysis Research Group, Neuropsychopharmacology Program, IMIM-
Hospital del Mar, carrer Dr. Aiguader 88, 08003 Barcelona, Spain

Thomas W. Storer
Section of Endocrinology, Diabetes, and Nutrition,
Boston University School of Medicine, Boston MA, USA

Christian J. Strasburger
Charité - Universitätsmedizin, Division of Clinical Endocrinology,
Department of Medicine, Campus Mitte , Berlin, Germany

Antoine Tabarin
Department of Endocrinology, CHU Haut-Lévêque, Pessac 33604, France

Arthur Weltman
Department of Human Services, University of Virginia, Charlottesville,
VA 22904, USA
and
Department of Medicine, University of Virginia, Charlottesville, VA 22904, USA
and
Exercise Physiology Program, University of Virginia, Charlottesville,
VA 22904, USA

Zida Wu
Division of Clinical Endocrinology, Charité – Universitätsmedizin Berlin,
Campus Mitte Berlin, Germany

Zvi Zadik
Chairman Research Authority, Kaplan Medical Center, Rehovot, Israel
and
School of Nutritional Sciences, Hebrew University, Rehovot, Israel

Michael Zitzmann
Centre for Reproductive Medicine and Andrology/Clinical Andrology,
University Clinics Müenster, Müenster, Germany

Mario Zorzoli
UCI Doctor and Scientific Adviser International Cycling Union,
Aigle, Switzerland

Chapter 1
GH/IGF-I Axis in Exercise

Enrico Gabellieri, Ignacio Bernabeu, Eva Fernandez, Monica Marazuela, Luca Chiovato, and Felipe F. Casanueva

Introduction

Growth hormone (GH) is secreted by the somatotrope cells of the anterior pituitary in a pulsatile manner. GH secretion is regulated by three peptides: growth hormone releasing hormone (GHRH), somatostatin, and growth hormone releasing peptide/ ghrelin. The two hypothalamic peptides, GHRH and somatostatin, exert an opposite effect on the somatotrope cells; indeed GHRH stimulates whereas somatostatin inhibits GH synthesis and secretion. Ghrelin, a peptide derived primarily from the endocrine cells of the stomach, stimulates GH release both directly and sinergistically with GHRH. GH interacts with 2 GH receptors (GHR) at two different binding sites, this interaction activates a signaling cascade of events resulting in the generation, mainly at hepatic level, of the insulin-like-growth-factor I (IGF-I) that regulates, through a feedback mechanism, GH release [1, 2]. Other factors can also modulate GH secretion, these include age, gender, nutritional state, sleep, body composition, stress, hormones (corticoids, gonadal steroids, thyroid hormones, insulin), and physical exercise [1]. Among these factors, acute physical exercise is a well-known potent stimulus to GH release [3].

Physiological Role of the GH-IGF-I Axis During Exercise

The GH-IGF-I axis shows widespread metabolic and biological effects. Among these actions the anabolic and lypolitic effects of GH are probably the most important during exercise. GH, directly and via IGF-I, increases protein synthesis and decreases protein catabolism by mobilizing fat as a principal fuel source.

E. Gabellieri (✉)
Fondazione Salvatore Maugeri Istituto di Ricovero e Cura a Carattere Scientifico, Chair of Endocrinology, University of Pavia, Via S. Maugeri 10, 27100 Pavia, Italy
e-mail: endocrine@usc.es

E. Ghigo et al. (eds.), *Hormone Use and Abuse by Athletes*, Endocrine Updates 29, DOI 10.1007/978-1-4419-7014-5_1, © Springer Science+Business Media, LLC 2011

Although several studies have investigated the physiological role of the GH-IGF-I axis during exercise, the contribution of GH to exercise capacity in normal subjects remains unclear. Indeed, the physiological mechanisms through which GH secretion increases during exercise and the exact neuroendocrine pathways that regulate GH secretion during exercise are still poorly understood although there is some evidence that adrenergic, cholinergic, and opioid pathways may be involved in this process [1]. Changes in body temperature [4], blood lactate levels [5] and pH [6] are supposed to play a role in the exercise stimulated GH rise. In particular, the fact that GH response to exercise is attenuated in the cold and is proportional to the core body temperature support a remarkable role of body temperature in the regulation of GH secretion during exercise [7].

Our current knowledge about the relationship between GH and exercise derives from studies conducted both in normal/athletes subjects and in growth hormone deficient (GHD) or acromegalic patients.

Evidences Derived from GHD Patients

In GHD patients the exercise performance, evaluated by the maximum ability to take in and use oxygen (VO_{2max}), by the ventilatory threshold (VeT) and by the maximal power output, is reduced. GH replacement therapy can improve and normalize all these parameters of exercise performance [8, 9]. Although not all the studies [10, 11] have demonstrated an improvement of the exercise capacity after GH replacement therapy, a recent metaanalysis [12] has shown positive and significant effect of GH replacement on overall exercise capacity.

Several mechanisms may explain the GH-induced improvement of exercise performance in GHD patients: increased delivery of substrate and oxygen to exercising muscle, increased fat oxidation with glycogen sparing, increased muscle strength, a combination of all these actions. Indirect mechanism, including changes in body composition or more efficient thermoregulation, could also exert a role in the improvement of exercise performance. GH and IGF-I have cardiorespiratory and hematological effects that can improve exercise capacity by increasing the delivery of substrate and oxygen to the exercising muscle. Indeed, in GHD patients, GH replacement therapy increases erythropoiesis [13], plasma volume, cardiac contractility [14], and probably reduces systemic vascular resistance [15]. Furthermore, GH can influence body fat, extracellular water, sweating and thermoregulation, all factors that affect the exercise capacity. In spite of all these actions, the relevance to exercise performance of the GH-IGF-I axis is mainly due to its metabolic effects. GH exerts an important metabolic role through its physiologically anabolic, lypolitic, and natriuretic actions. GH and IGF-I exert anabolic effects on skeletal muscle and this results in an increased muscle strength [16]. The anabolic effect of GH on protein metabolism during exercise is partially due to an increased fatty acids availability. Indeed, the most prominent metabolic effect of GH during exercise seems to be a marked increase in lipolysis and free fatty acids (FFAs) levels. FFAs represent an important metabolic fuel during exercise of medium and long duration; therefore, the GH response to exercise is important in the regulation of substrate availability and use during exercise [17]. It was observed that GH increases after the beginning of exercise and that this increase precedes the rise in FFAs plasma levels. There is also evidence suggesting that GH secretion could exert an immediate and also a delayed effect to increase FFAs availability after exercise. The fact that the increased lipolysis during exercise precedes the surge of GH secretion and that a GH pulse exerts a delayed effect to stimulate lypolisis under resting condition has lead to hypothesize that the main effect of the acute postexercise GH increase on lypolisis occurs in the postexercise period or during very prolonged exercise [18]. It is possible that this effect contributes to the changes in body composition and exercise performance occurring as a result of continuous training.

Variables that Influence GH Release During Exercise

Although exercise stimulates GH release, it is important to consider that different variables can influence the magnitude of this response in normal subjects (Fig. 1.1). Indeed, intensity, nature and duration of the exercise, physical fitness, gender, age, and body composition influence the GH response to exercise. GH levels start to increase 10–20 min after the onset of exercise, with a peak either at the end or shortly after exercise, and remain elevated for up to 2 h after exercise [19]. In younger men and women a linear dose–response relationship is observed between exercise intensity and GH release [20]. The increased GH levels result from an increase in the amount of GH secreted per pulse, with no change in pulse frequency or in the half life of elimination. GH secretion correlates positively with duration of exercise when intensity is constant [21], it is augmented by repetitive bouts of exercise [22] but is not influenced by the time of day in which exercise is performed [23]. Although both

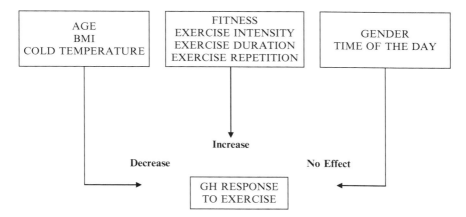

Fig. 1.1 Variables that can influence GH response to exercise

aerobic and resistance exercise result in significant increase in GH secretion, different exercise stimuli produce different GH response. Endurance exercise elicits a greater GH response than sprint and resistance exercise [24]. The comparison of GH secretion in men and in women [25], at rest and during exercise, shows that the GH secretion rate under resting condition is greater in women, but during exercise the increment from baseline is similar in men and women and does not correlate with sex hormones. The GH response to exercise is blunted with aging. Even in early middle age the GH response to exhaustive exercise is greatly attenuated compared with younger subjects [26]. The GH secretory rates are also reduced in overweight and obese subjects [27–29]. In particular, with aging, in spite of a physiological increase of body fat, the GH response has been found to be determined by age and physical fitness, as assessed by VO_{2max} but not by body fat [30].

Exercise exerts acute affects on other components of the GH/IGF-I axis. The GH-binding protein, total IGF-I, IGF binding protein (IGFBP)-3, and acid-labile subunit increase slightly during exercise, whereas IGFBP-1 secretion is enhanced by physical effort [31, 32]. Free IGF-I does not appear to change during or after exercise [33]. The pathophysiological relevance of these effects is not known, but it has been postulated that the modest increase in IGF-I might enhance postexercise reparative processes, or that the increased IGFBP-I levels might protect against delayed onset hypoglycaemia.

Supraphysiological GH Levels and Exercise Performance

The effects of supraphysiological GH administration on the metabolic response to exercise, on protein metabolism and muscle mass have also been investigated [34]. In this condition, GH seems to enhance lipolysis during exercise while sparing protein. Although, supraphysiological plasma GH levels can produce changes in body composition and an increase in muscle mass and strength, there is a lack of evidence that GH can be effective at improving exercise performance or endurance in athletes [35]. A useful model to study the chronic effect of GH excess is represented by acromegaly. Acromegaly is characterized by abnormalities in protein and carbohydrate metabolism and by impairments in strength and exercise performance. In particular, despite an increase in muscle mass, muscle fibers reveal a myopathic process producing in some patients an hypertrophy of type 1 and an atrophy of type 2 fibers [36]. The aerobic exercise capacity and cardiac performance are also impaired in acromegalic patients. The administration of supraphysiological doses of GH can produce different effects in normal young subjects as compared to athletes, elderly people or obese patients because in these subjects the GH secretion rates are very different. Thus, although there is little scientific evidence that in athletes the metabolic actions of supraphysiologic GH can improve exercise performance, some data suggest that GH treatment can improve body composition and exercise performance in elderly subjects, but at present, there are no evidences that GH can improve physical performance in obese subjects [37].

Conclusion

Data in the literature support the concept that an intact GH-IGF-I axis plays an important role in maintaining a normal exercise capacity. The GH response to exercise through the regulation of FFA availability can contribute to the exercise performance and to the anabolic effect of exercise. However, GH administration produces different effects in relation to a normal, increased or decreased GH and IGF-I production. Therefore, it is very important, when considering a possible GH treatment, to balance the effectiveness and the safety of this therapy.

References

1. Giustina A, Veldhuis JD. Pathophysiology of the neuroregulation of growth hormone secretion in experimental animals and the human. Endocr Rev. 1998; 19: 717–797.
2. Veldhuis JD. A tripeptidyl ensemble perspective of interactive control of growth hormone secretion. Horm Res. 2003; 60 (Suppl 1): 86–101.
3. Sutton J, Lazarus L. Growth hormone in exercise: comparison of physiological and pharmacological stimuli. J Appl Physiol. 1976; 41: 523–527.
4. Christensen SE, Jørgensen OL, Møller N, Orskov H. Characterization of growth hormone release in response to external heating. Comparison to exercise induced release. Acta Endocrinol (Copenh). 1984; 107: 295–301.
5. Felsing NE, Brasel JA, Cooper DM. Effect of low and high intensity exercise on circulating growth hormone in men. J Clin Endocrinol Metab. 1992; 75: 157–162.
6. Elias AN, Wilson AF, Naqvi S, Pandian MR. Effects of blood pH and blood lactate on growth hormone, prolactin, and gonadotropin release after acute exercise in male volunteers. Proc Soc Exp Biol Med. 1997; 214: 156–160.
7. Wheldon A, Savine RL, Sönksen PH, Holt RI. Exercising in the cold inhibits growth hormone secretion by reducing the rise in core body temperature. Growth Horm IGF Res. 2006; 16: 125–131.
8. Nass R, Huber RM, Klauss V, Müller OA, Schopohl J, Strasburger CJ. Effect of growth hormone (hGH) replacement therapy on physical work capacity and cardiac and pulmonary function in patients with hGH deficiency acquired in adulthood. J Clin Endocrinol Metab. 1995; 80: 552–557.
9. Whitehead HM, Boreman C, McIlrath EM, Sheridan B, Kennedy L, Atkinson AB, Hadden DR Growth hormone treatment of adults with growth hormone deficiency: results of a 13-month placebo controlled cross-over study. Clin Endocrinol (Oxf). 1992; 36: 45–52.
10. Beshyah SA, Freemantle C, Shahi M, Anyaoku V, Merson S, Lynch S, Skinner E, Sharp P, Foale R, Johnston DG. Replacement treatment with biosynthetic human growth hormone in growth hormone-deficient hypopituitary adults. Clin Endocrinol (Oxf). 1995; 42: 73–84.
11. Degerblad M, Almkvist O, Grunditz R, Hall K, Kaijser L, Knutsson E, Ringertz H, Thorén M. Physical and psychological capabilities during substitution therapy with recombinant growth hormone in adults with growth hormone deficiency. Acta Endocrinol (Copenh). 1990; 123: 185–193.
12. Widdowson WM, Gibney J. The effect of growth hormone replacement on exercise capacity in patients with GH deficiency: a metaanalysis. J Clin Endocrinol Metab. 2008; 93: 4413–4417.
13. Golde DW, Bersch N, Li CH. Growth hormone: species-specific stimulation of erythropoiesis in vitro. Science. 1977; 196: 1112–1113.
14. Saccà L, Cittadini A, Fazio S. Growth hormone and the heart. Endocr Rev. 1994; 15: 555–573.

15. Johannsson G, Sverrisdóttir YB, Ellegård L, Lundberg PA, Herlitz H. GH increases extracellular volume by stimulating sodium reabsorption in the distal nephron and preventing pressure natriuresis. J Clin Endocrinol Metab. 2002; 87: 1743–1749.
16. Janssen YJ, Doornbos J, Roelfsema F. Changes in muscle volume, strength, and bioenergetics during recombinant human growth hormone (GH) therapy in adults with GH deficiency. J Clin Endocrinol Metab. 1999; 84: 279–284.
17. Hunter WM, Fonseka CC, Passmore R. The role of growth hormone in the mobilization of fuel for muscular exercise. Q J Exp Physiol Cogn Med Sci. 1965; 50: 406–416.
18. Wee J, Charlton C, Simpson H, Jackson NC, Shojaee-Moradie F, Stolinski M, Pentecost C, Umpleby AM. GH secretion in acute exercise may result in post-exercise lipolysis. Growth Horm IGF Res. 2005; 15: 397–404.
19. Lassarre C, Girard F, Durand J, Raynaud J. Kinetics of human growth hormone during submaximal exercise. J Appl Physiol. 1974; 37: 826–830.
20. Pritzlaff-Roy CJ, Widemen L, Weltman JY, Abbott R, Gutgesell M, Hartman ML, Veldhuis JD, Weltman A. Gender governs the relationship between exercise intensity and growth hormone release in young adults. J Appl Physiol. 2002; 92: 2053–2060.
21. Wideman L, Consitt L, Patrie J, Swearingin B, Bloomer R, Davis P, Weltman A. The impact of sex and exercise duration on growth hormone secretion. J Appl Physiol. 2006; 101: 1641–1647.
22. Kanaley JA, Weltman JY, Veldhuis JD, Rogol AD, Hartman ML, Weltman A. Human growth hormone response to repeated bouts of aerobic exercise. J Appl Physiol. 1997; 83: 1756–1761.
23. Kanaley JA, Weltman JY, Pieper KS, Weltman A, Hartman ML. Cortisol and growth hormone responses to exercise at different times of day. J Clin Endocrinol Metab. 2001; 86: 2881–2889.
24. Gilbert KL, Stokes KA, Hall GM, Thompson D. Growth hormone responses to 3 different exercise bouts in 18- to 25- and 40- to 50-year-old men. Appl Physiol Nutr Metab. 2008; 33: 706–712.
25. Wideman L, Weltman JY, Shah N, Story S, Veldhuis JD, Weltman A. Effects of gender on exercise-induced growth hormone release. J Appl Physiol. 1999; 87: 1154–1162.
26. Zaccaria M, Varnier M, Piazza P, Noventa D, Ermolao A. Blunted growth hormone response to maximal exercise in middle aged versus young subjects and no effect of endurance training. J Clin Endocrinol Metab. 1999; 84: 2303–2307.
27. Veldhuis JD, Liem AY, South S, Weltman A, Weltman J, Clemmons DA, Abbott R, Mulligan T, Johnson ML, Pincus S. Differential impact of age, sex steroid hormones, and obesity on basal versus pulsatile growth hormone secretion in men as assessed in an ultrasensitive chemiluminescence assay. J Clin Endocrinol Metab. 1995; 80: 3209–3222.
28. Prange Hansen A. Serum growth hormone response to exercise in non-obese and obese normal subjects. Scand J Clin Lab Invest. 1973; 31: 175–178.
29. Scacchi M, Valassi E, Ascoli P, Cavagnini F. Obesity, hyponutrition and growth hormone. Obes Metab. 2007; 3: 68–87.
30. Holt RI, Webb E, Pentecost C, Sönksen PH. Aging and physical fitness are more important than obesity in determining exercise- induced generation of GH. J Clin Endocrinol Metab. 2001; 86: 5715–5720.
31. Bang P, Brandt J, Degerblad M, Enberg G, Kaijser L, Thorén M, Hall K. Exercise-induced changes in insulin-like growth factors and their low molecular weight binding protein in healthy subjects and patients with growth hormone deficiency. Eur J Clin Invest. 1990; 20: 285–292.
32. Schwarz AJ, Brasel JA, Hintz RL, Mohan S, Cooper DM. Acute effect of brief low- and high-intensity exercise on circulating insulin-like growth factor (IGF) I, II, and IGF-binding protein-3 and its proteolysis in young healthy men. J Clin Endocrinol Metab. 1996; 81: 3492–3497.
33. Wallace JD, Cuneo RC, Baxter R, Orskov H, Keay N, Pentecost C, Dall R, Rosén T, Jørgensen JO, Cittadini A, Longobardi S, Sacca L, Christiansen JS, Bengtsson BA, Sönksen PH. Responses of the growth hormone (GH) and insulin-like growth factor axis to exercise, GH administration, and GH withdrawal in trained adult males: a potential test for GH abuse in sport. J Clin Endocrinol Metab. 1999; 84: 3591–3601.
34. Healy ML, Gibney J, Pentecost C, Croos P, Russell-Jones DL, Sönksen PH, Umpleby AM. Effects of high-dose growth hormone on glucose and glycerol metabolism at rest and during exercise in endurance-trained athletes. J Clin Endocrinol Metab. 2006; 91: 320–327.

35. Berggren A, Ehrnborg C, Rosén T, Ellegård L, Bengtsson BA, Caidahl K. Short-term administration of supraphysiological recombinant human growth hormone (GH) does not increase maximum endurance exercise capacity in healthy, active young men and women with normal GH-insulin-like growth factor I axes. J Clin Endocrinol Metab. 2005; 90: 3268–3273.
36. Nagulesparen M, Trickey R, Davies MJ, Jenkins JS. Muscle changes in acromegaly. Br Med J. 1976; 16: 914–915.
37. Gibney J, Healy ML, Sönksen PH. The growth hormone/insulin-like growth factor-I axis in exercise and sport. Endocr Rev. 2007; 28: 603–624.

Chapter 2
Exercise, Training, and the Hypothalamo–Pituitary–Adrenal Axis

Martin Duclos and Antoine Tabarin

Activation of the HPA Axis During an Acute Bout of Exercise

During exercise, the HPA axis responds to numerous stimuli demonstrating the regulatory and integrative functions of the HPA axis: neuronal homeostatic signals (chemoreceptors, baroreceptors, and osmoreceptors stimulation), circulating homeostatic signals (glucose, leptin, atrial natriuretic peptide), and inflammatory signals (IL1, IL6, TNFa) [1]. In humans, the dynamics of the HPA axis activation during exercise associate stimulation of hypothalamic corticotropin-releasing hormone (CRH) and arginin-vasopressin (AVP) secretion (with a prominent role of CRH), and synthesis and release of ACTH from pituitary corticotroph cells preceding the increase of cortisol [2].

Two major factors modulate the HPA axis response to exercise: intensity and duration of exercise [3]. The minimum intensity of exercise (i.e., threshold) necessary to produce a cortisol response from the HPA axis is 60% of VO_2 max. Above 60% VO_2 max, a linear increase between the intensity of exercise and the increase in plasma cortisol concentrations is observed [4–6]. Below this intensity threshold, i.e., during light and prolonged exercise (<60% VO_2 max), ACTH and cortisol concentration may increase, with a duration threshold around 90 min of exercise at 40% VO_2 max [4]. These thresholds are independent of training. Indeed, when exercise is realized at similar relative intensity (%VO_2 max) between sedentary and trained men, the thresholds of intensity and duration for exercise-induced cortisol secretion are similar between the two groups as also the magnitude and duration of cortisol increase [4, 7–9].

Other factors can modulate the cortisol response to exercise such as hypohydration, meals, and time of day. Independently of external thermal stress, hypohydration (up to 4.8% body mass loss) potently amplifies the exercise-induced responses of cortisol to exercise. This enhancement of exercise-induced stress probably results from an increased core temperature and cardiovascular demand consecutive to decreased plasma volume [10]. Meals also stimulate cortisol release in humans. Exercise

A. Tabarin (✉)
Department of Endocrinology, CHU Haut-Lévêque, Pessac 33604, France
e-mail: antoine.tabarin@chu-bordeaux.fr

E. Ghigo et al. (eds.), *Hormone Use and Abuse by Athletes*, Endocrine Updates 29,
DOI 10.1007/978-1-4419-7014-5_2, © Springer Science+Business Media, LLC 2011

performed immediately after food ingestion results in a blunted cortisol response to the exercise stimulus, and conversely, the postprandial increase in serum cortisol concentrations is attenuated by prior exercise [11]. Finally, as the cortisol response to exercise is significantly modulated by time of day, neglecting the circadian cortisol variations may introduce errors into conclusion about the hormone responses to exercise and training [12, 13]. More specifically, the incremental response of cortisol to exercise is enhanced during the evening compared to morning exercise.

When repeated daily bouts of exercise are performed, the recovery time between bouts may also influence the HPA response to exercise. In male elite endurance athletes, the repetition of a prolonged strenuous exercise (bout of 75 min of exercise at 75% VO_2 max) induces a more pronounced increase in ACTH and cortisol when the previous bout of exercise was performed 3 h as opposed to 6 h earlier. This enhancement of the HPA axis activity during repetition of exercise occurs despite completely normalized plasma concentrations of cortisol and ACTH between the two exercise sessions. Thus, the duration of rest between the first and second sessions of exercise is a significant determinant of the magnitude of the cortisol response during reactivation of the HPA axis by the second bout of exercise [14]. These data must be considered in the light of the role of cortisol in consolidating glycogen reserve in muscle tissue, shutting off muscle inflammatory reaction and preparing the organism for the next bout of exercise [1]. Finally, whatever the type and the duration of exercise, plasma cortisol levels decrease to preexercise values within 120 min after the end of exercise [4, 7, 8, 12, 15, 16].

Adaptation of the HPA Axis to Endurance-Training

According to the data mentioned above, an exercise such as a 2-h run induces an increase in cortisol concentrations for at least 3 h (the second hour of exercise and the 2 h of postexercise recovery) (Fig. 2.1) [7]. When training for a marathon race, subjects run an average of 120–180 km/week. This implies daily sessions of prolonged and/or intense running and consequently prolonged phases of endogenous hypercortisolism (i.e., during exercise and during postimmediate exercise recovery). These periods of hypercortisolism are mandatory for fuel mobilization that is needed to achieve prolonged and/or intense exercise. However, given the antagonistic action of GC on muscle anabolic processes and their immunosuppressive effects, we have hypothesized that endurance-trained men may develop adaptive mechanisms such as decreased sensitivity to cortisol to protect muscle against this cortisol oversecretion. Through these adaptive processes, the HPA axis may cope with repeated stimulations, allowing, on the one hand, the ability of the organism to respond adequately to repeated stimulations and, on the other hand, protecting some GC sensitive tissues from high cortisol levels.

Since the last decade, several studies have shown that in endurance-trained subjects, 24 h cortisol secretion is not increased *under nonexercising conditions*. Accordingly, 800 h plasma cortisol, nycthemeral cortisol rhythm, overnight and 24 h urinary free

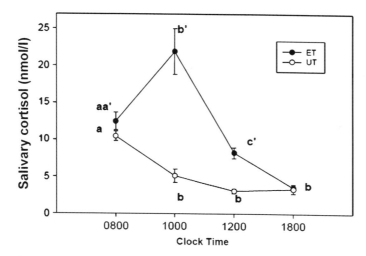

Fig. 2.1 Saliva cortisol concentrations across time during the experimental day in endurance-trained (ET) men (exercise and resting sessions) and untrained (UT) men (resting session). ET men realized a 2-h run between 800 and 1,000 h. *Bars* not sharing a common letter are significantly different from each others. Results are means ± sem. From Duclos et al. [8]. At 800 h, saliva cortisol concentrations were similar between UT and ET men. Two hours of exercise induced an increase of cortisol at the end of exercise (1,000 h) and 2 h after the end of exercise (1,200 h) (ET)

cortisol (UFC), seasonal rhythmicity of cortisol excretion, and cortisol response to dexamethasone suppression test in resting endurance-trained subjects are similar to those of age-matched sedentary subjects [4, 9, 12, 15]. Altogether, these results probe the functional integrity of the HPA axis in endurance-trained subjects. The overactivity of the HPA axis reported by some authors [5, 17] may represent a further step in the intensity of physical activity strain, leading to overreaching and/or overtraining and pathological adaptations of the HPA axis. As suggested by Luger et al. [5], the highly trained group of people that they studied and who presented with mild evening hypercortisolism may have included subjects whose personalities had anorectic or depressive components, all conditions associated with chronic activation of the HPA axis. In women, alterations of the HPA axis in amenorrheic runners have been reported, with UFC levels elevated to levels observed in anorexia nervosa [17]. However, the physiopathology of this increased cortisol secretion has been extensively explained by De Souza and Loucks [18, 19], who repeatedly demonstrated that it is the stress of chronic energy deficiency (negative energy balance) that induces this chronic hypercortisolism and not the stress of exercise by itself.

Contrary to their apparently similar resting HPA axis activity, endurance-trained subjects differ from sedentary subjects when their HPA axis is challenged. These differences are highlighted when the HPA axis function is evaluated during the immediate postexercise recovery period (when plasma cortisol is still increased) and can be summarized as follows (Fig. 2.1). During this critical period and despite postexercise increased plasma cortisol concentrations, the HPA axis of trained subjects is still able to respond to subsequent physiological (food intake [4], exercise [4, 14]) or pharmacological challenges (ACTH 250 μg [20], CRF/LVP test [20]). This ability to respond to a second stimulation during this critical period is not observed in sedentary subjects. These results suggest a decreased pituitary sensitivity to the early GC negative feedback in endurance-trained athletes. The cortisol response to food intake illustrates this difference. In sedentary men, Brandenberger et al. [11] have shown that the daily cortisol pattern results from the interactions between the meal-related peaks, especially the major midday cortisol peak, and the exercise-induced cortisol increases, both of which inhibit the responses to subsequent stimulation. It explains why in conditions of exercise-induced marked cortisol increase, the subsequent stimulation exerted by meal taken 1 h after a 2-h run did not elicit a rise of cortisol levels in sedentary men [4]. By contrast, endurance-trained men, despite similar increased cortisol concentrations, are able to escape to the blunting effect of the preceding exercise-induced cortisol increase (GC feedback), and therefore, to respond to subsequent stimulation with a significant cortisol increase to noon meal [4].

Different mechanisms can be involved in this adaptation. At the level of the central nervous system, neuropeptides and corticosteroid receptors (GR, MR) in the brain and anterior pituitary play a major role in the regulation of circulating cortisol levels. The influence of exercise on these central regulators in humans is largely unexplored for evident methodological reasons. In animals, studies investigating the mechanisms underlying the potential influence of exercise training on the central regulation of HPA axis activity have used forced exercise protocols (treadmill training or swimming) [21]. In rats and mice, forced exercise induces different regulatory changes in the HPA axis compared to voluntary exercise (allowing access to a running wheel in the cage) and must be regarded as a chronic stress paradigm. Using voluntary access to a running wheel, Droste et al. [21] have shown that long-term (4 weeks) exercising mice showed unchanged GR levels, whereas MR levels were decreased in hippocampus of exercising animals. CRH mRNA levels in the paraventricular nucleus were also lower in exercising mice. Thus, voluntary exercise in rodents resulted in complex adaptive changes at various levels within the HPA axis and limbic/neocortical efferent control mechanisms.

At the peripheral level, tissular sensitivity to GC may also be different between endurance-trained and sedentary subjects. Changes in availability and/or sensitivity to GC may explain the apparent discrepancy between repeated and prolonged exercise-induced HPA axis activation (during exercise and 1–2 h postexercise) and the lack of metabolic consequences of such increased cortisol secretion. Duclos et al. [8] have reported an in vitro plasticity of monocytes sensitivity to GC in endurance-trained men, superimposed to changes in systemic cortisol concentrations. Despite similar resting cortisol levels, the sensitivity of monocytes to GC in endurance-trained men is decreased 8 and 24 h after the end of the last training session compared to sedentary men (Fig. 2.2). However, an acute bout of exercise increased the sensitivity of monocytes to GC of such endurance-trained subjects to the level observed in untrained men (Fig. 2.2). This transient decreased sensitivity of monocytes to GC in endurance-trained men may be related to a process of desensitization, which is supposed to protect the body from long-lasting exercise-induced

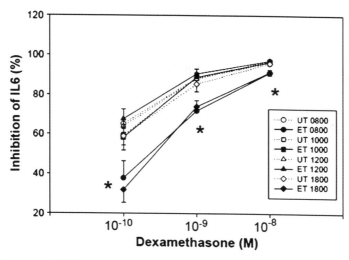

Fig. 2.2 Percentage inhibition of lipopolysaccharide (LPS) (0.3 µg/ml)-stimulated IL-6 production in cultures of peripheral monocytes in ET (*solid lines*) and UT men (*dotted lines*). *Asterisk*: The percent values of dexamethasone-induced IL-6 inhibition are significantly lower in ET at 800 and 1,800 h as compared with their values at 1,000 and 1,200 h, and as compared with the values of UT men at 800, 1,000, 1,200, and 1,800 h ($p<0.05$). From Duclos et al. [8]. The sensitivity to glucocorticoids (GC) in UT men is similar at every time sampling between 800 and 1,800 h, despite different plasma cortisol levels (Fig. 2.1). At 800 h, monocytes of ET men were less sensitive to dexamethasone than those from UT men. An acute exercise (between 800 and 1,000 h) increased the sensitivity of monocytes to GC in ET men to the levels observed in control ET men

cortisol secretion. However, this observation should not be generalized to the whole organism since differences in GC sensitivity across tissues (immune system, cardiovascular system, and the HPA axis) have been shown in healthy subjects [22].

Upstream these cellular mechanisms, the extracellular and/or the intracellular availability of cortisol could also be modified. Extracellular bioavailability depends on the free fraction of cortisol. Cortisol largely binds to plasma proteins and especially to the cortisol-binding globulin (CBG). Thus, plasma cortisol levels are modulated by variations of CBG and poorly correlate with cortisol production rates unless differences in CBG are corrected [3]. Saliva cortisol concentrations closely reflect the free – active – plasma cortisol [3]. Measuring simultaneously plasma and saliva cortisol concentrations, we did not find differences in endurance-trained men vs. sedentary men, in resting conditions as well as during exercise [7–9, 23]. In addition to CBG which modulates the extracellular availability of cortisol, the access of cortisol to target cells is controlled by prereceptor metabolism of cortisol. Tissue-specific enzymes 11β hydroxysteroid dehydrogenases (11β-HSD), which interconvert hormonally active cortisol and inactive cortisone, have been shown to modulate cortisol hormone action in several peripheral tissues [24]. The crucial physiological principle illuminated by the action of 11β-HSD is that cortisol action on target cells is determined by enzyme activity within the cells, rather than circulating cortisol levels alone. Interestingly, the 24-h urinary cortisol/cortisone ratio (an index of whole body 11β-HSD activity [25]) was reported to be negatively related to the total training load in a population of swimmers [26]. This suggests that any significant increase in 24-h cortisol secretion is balanced by its parallel inactivation into cortisone. Elsewhere, the nocturnal period is essential for exercise recovery. Gouarne et al. [9] have studied the overnight GC output to assess the delicate balance between cumulative fatigue resulting from exercise training and its recovery period over a 10-month season in triathletes. To dissociate the effects of training from those of seasonal hormonal variations, endurance-trained men were compared to sedentary men [9]. Gouarne et al. reported similar overnight urinary cortisol output in both groups during the 10-month follow-up. Moreover, whereas overnight urinary cortisol excretion showed seasonal variations (November > June) in both groups, urinary cortisol/cortisone excretion remained stable in both groups during the follow-up period, suggesting again that any significant increase in cortisol secretion (seasonal-induced increased cortisol secretion) is balanced by its parallel inactivation into cortisone. The importance of this mechanism is also highlighted in the two triathletes of this study who developed an overtraining syndrome (decreased performance, high score of fatigue, and inability to maintain the training load) during the follow-up: both presented a sharp decrease of inactivation of cortisol into cortisone with increased cortisol/cortisone ratio compared to their basal (pretraining values) and compared to the values of the other triathletes at the same period.

In conclusion, endurance-training subjects have similar HPA axis activity in resting condition than healthy sedentary subjects. However, when the HPA axis is challenged, endurance-trained subjects demonstrate a decreased pituitary (and probably hypothalamic and/or suprahypothalamic) sensitivity to the negative feedback of GC that explain their capacity to achieve successfully a second bout of exercise separated by a short rest period. Successful adaptation to exercise-induced repeated and prolonged cortisol secretion also includes decreased peripheral tissue sensitivity to GC that is supposed to protect the body from the severe metabolic and immune consequences of increased cortisol levels. A great diversity of mechanisms is involved in such adaptation, acting at potentially all levels in the cascade leading to the biological effects of cortisol.

References

1. Sapolsky RM, Romero M, Munck AU. How do glucocorticoids influence stress responses? Integrating permissive, suppressive, stimulatory, and preparative actions. Endocr Rev. 2000; 21:55–89.
2. Smoak B, Deuster PA, Rabin D, Chrousos GP. Corticotropin-releasing hormone is not the sole factor mediating exercise-induced adrenocorticotropin release in humans. J Clin Endocrinol Metab. 1991; 73:302–306.
3. Duclos M, Guinot M, Le Bouc Y. Cortisol and GH: odd and controversial ideas. Appl Physiol Nutr Metab. 2007; 32(5):895–903.
4. Duclos M, Corcuff JB, Rashedi M, et al. Trained versus untrained men: different immediate post-exercise responses of pituitary-adrenal axis. Eur J Appl Physiol. 1997; 75:343–350.

5. Luger A, Deuster PA, Kyle SB, et al. Acute hypothalamic-pituitary-adrenal responses to the stress of treadmill exercise. New Engl J Med. 1987; 316:1309–1315.
6. Kjaer M, Secher NH, Bach FW, Galbo H. Role of motor center activity for hormonal changes and substrate mobilization in humans. Am J Physiol. 1987; 253:R687–R695.
7. Duclos M, Minkhar M, Sarrieau A, et al. Reversibility of endurance training-induced changes on glucocorticoid sensitivity of monocytes by an acute exercise. Clin Endocrinol. 1999; 51:749–756.
8. Duclos M, Gouarne C, Bonnemaison D. Acute and chronic effects of exercise on tissue sensitivity to glucocorticoids. J Appl Physiol. 2003; 94:869–875.
9. Gouarne C, Groussard C, Duclos M. Overnight urinary cortisol and cortisone add new insights into adaptation to training. Med Sci Sports Exerc. 2005; 37(7):1157–1167.
10. Judelson DA, Maresh CM, Yamamoto LM, et al. Effect of hydration state on resistance exercise-induced endocrine markers of anabolism, catabolism, and metabolism. J Appl Physiol. 2008; 105(3):816–824.
11. Brandenberger G, Follenius M, Hietter B, et al. Feedback from meal-related peaks determines diurnal changes in cortisol response to exercise. J Clin Endocrinol Metab. 1982; 54:592–594.
12. Kanaley JA, Weltman JY, Pieper KS, et al. Cortisol and growth hormone responses to exercise at different times of day. J Clin Endocrinol Metab. 2001; 86:2881–2889.
13. Thuma JR, Gilders R, Verdun M, Loucks AB. Circadian rhythm of cortisol confounds cortisol responses to exercise: implications for future research. J Appl Physiol. 1995; 78:1657–1664.
14. Ronsen O, Kjeldsen-Kragh J, Haug E, et al. Recovery time affects immunoendocrine responses to a second bout of endurance exercise. Am J Physiol. 2002; 283:C1612–C1620.
15. Kern W, Perras B, Wodick R, et al. Hormonal secretion during nighttime sleep indicating stress of daytime exercise. J Appl Physiol. 1995; 79:1461–1468.
16. Nindl BC, Friedl KE, Frykman PN, et al. Physical performance and metabolic recovery among lean, healthy men following a prolonged energy deficit. Int J Sports Med. 1997; 18:317–324.
17. Villanueva AL, Schlosser C, Hopper B, et al. Increased cortisol production in women runners. J Clin Endocrinol Metab. 1986; 63(1):133–136.
18. De Souza MJ, Van Heest J, Demers LM, Lasley BL. Luteal phase deficiency in recreational runners: evidence for a hypometabolic state. J Clin Endocrinol Metab. 2003; 88:337–346.
19. Loucks AB, Thuma JR. Luteinizing hormone pulsatility is disrupted at a threshold of energy availability in regularly menstruating women. J Clin Endocrinol Metab. 2003; 88:297–311.
20. Duclos M, Corcuff JB, Pehourcq F, Tabarin A. Decreased pituitary sensitivity to glucocorticoids in endurance trained men. Eur J Endocrinol. 2001; 144:363–368.
21. Droste SK, Gesing A, Ulbricht S, et al. Effects of long-term voluntary exercise on the mouse hypothalamic-pituitary-adrenocortical axis. Endocrinology. 2003; 144(7):3012–3023.
22. Ebrecht M, Buske-Kirschbaum A, Hellammer D, et al. Tissue specificity of glucocorticoid sensitivity in healthy adults. J Clin Endocrinol Metab. 2000; 85(10):3733–3739.
23. Duclos M, Corcuff JB, Arsac L, et al. Corticotroph axis sensitivity after exercise in endurance-trained athletes. Clin Endocrinol. 1998; 48:493–501.
24. Seckl JR, Walker BR. Minireview: 11b-hydroxysteroid dehydrogenase type 1 – a tissue specific amplifier of glucocorticoid action. Endocrinology. 2001; 142:1371–1376.
25. Best R, Walker BR. Additional value of measurement of urinary cortisone and unconjugated cortisol metabolites in assessing the activity of 11 beta-hydroxysteroid dehydrogenase in vivo. Clin Endocrinol (Oxf). 1997; 47(2):231–236.
26. Atlaoui D, Duclos M, Gouarne C, et al. The 24-h urinary cortisol/cortisone ratio for monitoring training in elite swimmers. Med Sci Sports Exerc. 2004; 36:218–224.

Chapter 3
Thyroid Axis, Prolactin, and Exercise

Anthony C. Hackney

Introduction

The endocrine system, from a classic biology perspective, is composed of a series of glandular tissues located throughout the human body, which secrete chemical substances (hormones) to modify/regulate the physiological function of target tissues. Many hormones not only have such endocrine effects, but also autocrine- and paracrine-like function. In the last few decades, many nonglandular tissues in the human body have been found to secrete hormonal agents (e.g., adipocytes → leptin) and hormonal-like substances such as cytokines (e.g., skeletal muscle → IL-6). Such discoveries have added to the complexity of trying to understand the endocrine-hormone controls in humans; but, such new and exciting findings have created a stimulating time to be an endocrinologist.

This chapter addresses some of the recent developments in our understanding of the thyroid hormones and the hormone prolactin. Contemporary research points to new, evolving and interactive roles for these hormones physiologically with respect to exercise and exercise training.

Thyroid Hormones

Physiological Function: Regulation

The thyroid gland is a highly critical endocrine gland in human. This gland secretes three hormones into the circulatory vascular bed, these are: thyroxine [3,5,3′,5′-tetraiodothyronine (T_4)], triiodothyronine [3,5,3′-triiodothyronine (T_3)], and calcitonin.

A.C. Hackney, Ph.D., D.Sc. (✉)
Applied Physiology Laboratory, Department of Exercise & Sport Science,
Department of Nutrition – School of Public Health, University of North Carolina,
Fetzer Building – CB # 8700, Chapel Hill, NC 27599-8700, USA
e-mail: ach@email.unc.edu

E. Ghigo et al. (eds.), *Hormone Use and Abuse by Athletes*, Endocrine Updates 29,
DOI 10.1007/978-1-4419-7014-5_3, © Springer Science+Business Media, LLC 2011

Both T_4 and T_3 are essential for normal physiological function within a board spectrum of tissues – organs, due to their ability to modulate metabolism and act in a synergistic fashion with other hormones. Conversely, calcitonin is a key regulator in maintaining the circulating levels of calcium, specifically via influence on osteoblastic-osteoclastic cellular activity and renal function. Due to space limitations, only T_4 and T_3 (collectively referred to as "thyroids" in this discussion) endocrine physiology are addressed here.

The glandular production/secretion of the thyroids is controlled by thyroid-stimulating hormone (TSH [i.e., thyrotropin]), a glycoprotein-based hormone released from the anterior pituitary (adenohypophysis). Thyroid-releasing hormone (TRH) produced by the hypothalamus stimulates the release of TSH. The control and release of these hormones involve a negative feedback loop referred to as the hypothalamic-pituitary-thyroidal axis [1, 2]. Table 3.1 lists those factors associated with stimulation-inhibition of the thyroid axis.

Once the thyroids are released into the circulation, these hormones exist in a bound as well as a free, unbound form. The carrier proteins for the bound forms of the hormones are: thyroid-binding globulin (TBG, accounting for 70%), thyroxine-binding

Table 3.1 Select factors associated with the regulatory control of thyroid axis and prolactin in humans

Hormone	Physiological regulatory factors
TRH	+ Norepinephrine + Sleep + Emotional-physical stress + Low ambient temperatures – Somatostatin (GHRH) – Dopamine
TSH	+ TRH + Estrogens – Growth hormone – Glucocorticoids
T_4 T_3	+ TSH – T_4 – T_3
Prolactin (Anterior pituitary source)	+ Emotional-physical stress + TRH + Insulin + Vasoactive intestinal polypeptide + Pregnancy lactation + Estrogens – Caloric deficiency – Dopamine
(Extra-pituitary source)	+ Local nucleotides – transcription factors (e.g., Activator protein-1, C/EBP, and CREB) + Catecholamines +/– Progesterone – IL-1β, IL-2, and IL-4

The [+] symbol indicates a stimulatory effect while the [−] symbol denotes an inhibitory effect pre-albumin (TBPA, 10–15%), and albumin (15–20%). The unbound free forms of T_4 and T_3 are relatively small amounts of each hormone's respective total amounts (free $T_4 \sim 0.03\%$; free $T_3 \sim 0.3\%$). These free forms are the most biologically active versions of each hormone [1].

In healthy individuals, circulating levels of T_4 exceed that of T_3, but T_3 is the most biologically potent of the two hormones. The turnover rate of the thyroids is very low relative to their existing large extracellular hormonal pool. This fact can make it complex and challenging for researchers to detect hormonal changes (even relatively large ones) in thyroid gland activity following a perturbation [1, 2].

Most tissues of the human body are strongly influenced metabolically by the thyroids. These hormones profoundly influence a multitude of tissue functions, growth, and development across the human life span [1, 3, 4]. For example, thyroids increase oxidative phosphorylation metabolism at the mitochondria and thus can elevate basal metabolic rate. They increase tissue responsiveness to the catecholamines (permissiveness), which can have a cardiogenic effect, increasing heart rate and contractility of the myocardium. The thyroids have a synergistic effect with growth hormone and thereby magnify the actions of this latter hormone. Furthermore, the thyroids facilitate the neuronal maturation process. They can also substantially augment lipid metabolism within the skeletal muscle as well as enhance hepatic glycogenolysis and in-turn impact blood glucose turnover rate [1, 2].

Exercise Effects on the Thyroid Hormones

Short-term incremental exercise (≤20 min) elevates blood TSH levels, with a critical intensity threshold of approximately ≥50% of maximal oxygen uptake (VO_{2max}) necessary to induce significant changes [3, 5]. Even though TSH is elevated, most research involving short-term exercise indicates that total and free T_4 and T_3 levels are not immediately affected [3]. Conversely, total T_4 and T_3 levels can increase following such exercise; however, these findings appear to be primarily brought about by exercise-induced hemoconcentration (i.e., many carrier proteins are trapped in the vascular space) [2, 6]. An increase in TSH would be expected to stimulate the thyroid gland and free hormone levels elevate, but there exist a delay inherent in the stimulus-secretion response of the gland [1]. Thus, if a blood sampling protocol is not extended long enough following exercise, thyroid changes are not detected. Regrettably, this procedural limitation seems to exist in many exercise research studies. Research findings are also compounded by the fact that in some situations the influential factors such as environment, dietary practices, and diurnal hormonal secretion patterns are not controlled effectively and thereby cannot be entirely separated from the influence of exercise alone [4, 7].

The influence of more prolonged submaximal exercise (approaching 60 min) on thyroids is controversial. Some investigations report no effect on blood TSH levels [3, 5, 8] while others have found that TSH and/or free T_3 [9] increase progressively with high intensity steady-state workloads and reach a steady-state elevated level by approximately 40 min of exercise [3, 5]. Berchtold et al. report that during very prolonged submaximal exercise (~3 h), total T_4 becomes elevated (constant) but then declines significantly following the exercise (i.e., in recovery) [8]. In the same study, the level of total T_3 was found to actually decline continuously during exercise. Conversely, Hackney and Gulledge found that total T_3 was unchanged, but total T_4 increased after 60 min of a prolonged steady-state submaximal exercise session [10]. On the other hand, Galbo [5] reports that highly strenuous, prolonged exercise to exhaustion increased only circulating free T_4 levels. Furthermore, Opstad [11] as well as others report that repeated days of stressful, demanding physical activity, substantially reduces T_4, T_3, and TSH levels [3]. These divergent findings are difficult to interpret due to the highly variable exercise sessions (i.e., different durations and intensities of exercise) and the varying blood sampling protocol employed [7].

Evidence suggests that intensive anaerobic exercise (cycling-interval training) increases total T_4 levels for several hours following the exercise, but not T_3 [3, 10]. These changes appear not due to hemoconcentration alone, but to what degree the changes are from increased T_4 secretion and/or a suppressed metabolic clearance rate (MCR) is unclear [7]. Research on the effects of resistance exercise, which tends to be anaerobic in nature, on the thyroids is sparse. McMurray and associates performed a well-controlled study looking at thyroids immediately after an intensive resistance-training session, as well as for 12 h into recovery (during the night time) from the exercise [6]. Transient but significant elevations in total T_4 and T_3 levels occurred immediately after exercise, apparently induced by hemoconcentration. However later, total T_3 level was significantly elevated nocturnally. These authors interpreted these changes as related to a thyroid-mediated increase in metabolism, most likely associated with tissue repairs and an increase in protein synthesis [1].

Research suggests that the effects of exercise training programs (chronic exposure) on thyroids are equivocal. Some studies (but not all) demonstrate that the rate of T_4 secretion is higher in exercise-trained individuals than in untrained individuals [3–5]. Blood levels of the hormone, however, are not elevated, suggesting a higher turnover rate for the hormone [12]. Conversely, Galbo [5] reports that a short-term, intensive exercise training periods result in significant reductions in the levels of select thyroids, a finding collaborated by others [13]. The discrepancy in the findings may be related to the fact that these studies failed to completely account for nutrient balance influences on thyroid turnover rate. That is, a negative energy balance has been shown to substantially reduce the thyroids [1, 2, 14]. However, Baylor and Hackney found that resting free T_3 and TSH are reduced during intensive competitive periods even when no significant changes in overall energy balance status occur [13]. As noted, the turnover rate of thyroid hormones appears to be increased in training athletes [3, 15], and perhaps as is the tissue sensitivity [1, 12, 15], which could account for the changes in thyroids noted above. Further work is warranted on this latter topic [16]. Finally, it is important to note that the exercise-induced change in free levels of the thyroids does not seem to change the capacity of binding proteins, either in response to acute or chronic exercise exposure [16, 17]. This suggests that either production/ secretion or MCR alterations are bringing about these changes.

Prolactin

Physiological Function: Regulation

In humans, the hormone prolactin is primarily secreted by the lactotrope cells of the adenohypophysis, but also it is secreted from the breast, the decidua, adipose tissue, parts of the central nervous system, and immune system. Because it is released by extra-pituitary sites, it is not only classified as a circulating hormone but also as an autocrine and paracrine factor. It is a multifunctional hormone, and many tissues within humans express prolactin receptors. Its release and physiological function has been linked to emotional-physical stress response, water balance regulation, fetal surfactant development, immune system activation, and reproductive function. A vast majority of the research on prolactin relates to this last topic due to the fact that prolactin has long been associated with lactogenesis in women and in excessive quantities to gonadal suppression in both men and women. The circulating levels of prolactin display a diurnal secretion pattern with peak levels during REM sleep [18].

The secretion of pituitary prolactin is under a constant inhibition via dopamine from the hypothalamus, but this inhibition can be over-ridden by certain physiological factors. Table 3.1 presents a brief listing of select factors associated with the stimulation and inhibition of prolactin.

Exercise Effects on Prolactin

Blood prolactin levels increase during exercise, with the magnitude of the increase approximately proportional to the intensity of the activity. Whether there is a critical intensity threshold necessary to induce a response is uncertain, but most exercise above the anaerobic threshold initiates substantial elevations in the hormone [3, 5, 19]. Provided the intensity is adequate, the increase in prolactin is quite rapid. Nonetheless, short-term, graded (incremental) exercise may result in a peak hormonal response occurring after the end of the exercise. In some situations, excessive emotional stress can cause an anticipatory increase in prolactin even before the beginning of exercise [3].

As for prolonged exercise, the prolactin response is proportional to the intensity at which it is performed. However, extending the duration of exercise can augment the magnitude of the prolactin response [20, 21]. This change in prolactin with prolonged exercise seems to be strongly driven by the elevation in core temperature in response to the exercise [22], and even just head-facial cooling has been shown to mitigate to some degree the prolactin response to such exercise [23]. Interestingly, during the night time, after a day-time bout of prolonged exercise, there is a two to three times increase in the nocturnal levels of the hormone [24].

Strenuous, high-intensive anaerobic exercise (cycling-intervals) results in greater prolactin responses than typically seen in submaximal aerobic exercise [25]. Unfortunately, the effect of resistance exercise on prolactin has not been extensively studied. Some evidence supports that this form of exercise will elevate prolactin, but the increase may occur actually after following the exercise session [3].

Data are contradictory with regard to the chronic effect of exercise training on basal, resting prolactin levels. Some studies have found an increase in resting levels, while others have found decreased levels [26, 27]. These contradictions are most likely related to differences in training protocols (intensity, frequency, and duration of training sessions). Hackney and associates have shown that the prolactin response to submaximal exercise in men is attenuated following training, but the maximal exercise response is augmented [3, 28]. Interestingly, in both men and women who have undergone a training program, the drug-stimulated prolactin response is enhanced (i.e., pituitary challenge tests [29, 30]). Why these somewhat disparate responses occur with regard to chronic exercise training is unclear and in need of further research.

Interaction of Thyroid Hormones and Prolactin

The thyroids and prolactin are inter-related more so than might initially appear, as they share certain aspects of regulation in common (see Table 3.1). A prime example of this is the fact that an increase in TRH release from the hypothalamus is not only a stimulant to the release of TSH, but also to the release of pituitary prolactin. In addition, estrogens provide an inter-connective regulatory link as they exert positive effects on the thyroids and prolactin. Likewise, "stressful" situations can result in TRH-TSH release as well as prolactin release [2, 18].

Hackney and Dobridge have demonstrated that this relationship between the thyroids and prolactin exists in response to exercise [31]. These authors found there were increases in TSH, free T_4, and free T_3 as well as prolactin immediately following intensive prolonged endurance exercise. The prolactin and thyroid responses were substantially related to one another (significant correlation analysis). It was speculated that the thyroid responses were being influenced by concurrent TRH changes, which also subsequently facilitated the corresponding prolactin changes.

One might wonder the utility of these inter-related responses during exercise or afterwards. Prolactin can be described, in general, as an immunopermissive hormone. Animal work supports that exercise prolactin increases are at levels elevated enough to stimulate chemotaxis, phagocytosis, and microbicidal capacity of phagocytes [18, 32]. Furthermore, prolactin can cause a dose-dependent inhibition of the release of the pro-inflammatory cytokine, interleukin-6 [18, 32]. Thyroids can also modulate macrophage function during exercise, specifically chemotaxis and phagocytosis [32]. Collectively, these findings suggest that the thyroids and prolactin may have roles, in concert, to aid and support the tissue inflammatory responses after exercise as part of the adaptive-regeneration process to exercise and exercise training [19, 33]. Future research needs to address this issue in detail and study the specifics of these fascinating hormonal interactions.

References

1. Griffin JE. The thyroid. In: Griffin JE & Odjeda SR (eds). Textbook of Endocrine Physiology, 3rd Edition. Oxford University: New York, pp. 260–283, 1996.
2. Mazzaferri EL. The thyroid. In: Mazzaferri, EL (ed). Endocrinology, 3rd Edition. Medical Examination Publishing Co.: New York, pp. 89–350, 1985.
3. McMurray RG & AC Hackney. The endocrine system and exercise. In: Garrett W, Kirkendahl D (eds). Exercise & Sports Science. Williams & Wilkins Publisher: New York, pp. 135–162, 2000.
4. McMurray RG & AC Hackney. Interactions of metabolic hormones, adipose tissue and exercise. Sports Med. 35(5): 393–412, 2005.
5. Galbo H. The hormonal response to exercise. Diabetes Metab Rev. 1(4): 385–408, 1986.
6. McMurray RG, TE Eubanks & AC Hackney. Nocturnal hormonal responses to weight training exercise. Eur J Appl Physiol. 72: 121–126, 1995.
7. Hackney AC & A Viru. Research methodology: issues with endocrinological measurements in exercise science and sport medicine. J Athletic Training. 43(6): 631–639, 2008.
8. Berchtold P, M Berger & HJ Uppers. Non-glucoregulatory hormones (T_4, T_3, rT_3 and testosterone) during physical exercise in juvenile type diabetes. Horm Metab Res. 10: 269–273, 1978.
9. Moore AW, S Timmerman, KK Brownlee, DA Rubin & AC Hackney. Strenuous, fatiguing exercise: relationship of cortisol to circulating thyroid hormones. Int J Endocrino Metab. 1: 18–24, 2005.
10. Hackney AC & TP Gulledge. Thyroid responses during an 8 hour period following aerobic and anaerobic exercise. Physiol Res. 43: 1–5, 1994.
11. Opstad K. Circadian rhythm of hormones is extinguished during prolonged physical stress, sleep and energy deficiency in young men. Eur J Endocrinol. 131(1): 56–66, 1994.
12. Irvine CHG. Effects of exercise on thyroxine degradation in athletes and non-athletes. J Clin Endocr. 28: 942–948, 1968.
13. Baylor LS & AC Hackney. Resting thyroid and leptin hormone changes in women following intense, prolonged exercise training. Eur J Appl Physiol. 88(4–5): 480–484, 2003.
14. Douyon L & DE Schteingart. Effect of obesity and starvation on thyroid hormone, growth hormone, and cortisol secretion. Endocrinol Metab Clin North Am. 31(1): 173–189, 2002.
15. Balsam A & LE Leppo. Effect of physical training on the metabolism of thyroid hormones in man. J Appl Physiol. 38: 212–215, 1975.
16. Terjung RL & WW Winder. Exercise and thyroid function. Med Sci Sports. 7(1): 20–26, 1974.
17. DeNayer P, M Ostyn & M DeVisscher. Effect de l'entrainement sur le taux de la thyroxine libre chez l'athlete. Annl D'Endocr. 31: 721–723, 1970.
18. Ben-Jonathan N, ER Hugo, TG Brandebourg & CR LaPensee. Focus on prolactin as a metabolic hormone. Trends Endocrinol. 17(3): 110–116, 2006.
19. Viru A & M Viru. Biochemical Monitoring of Sport Training. Human Kinetics Publishing, Champaign, IL, 2001.
20. Daly W, CA Seegers, DA Rubin, JD Dobridge & AC Hackney. Relationship between stress hormones and testosterone with prolonged endurance exercise. Eur J Appl Physiol. 93: 375–380, 2005.
21. Radomski MW, M Cross & A Buguet. Exercise-induced hyperthermia and hormonal responses to exercise. Can J Physiol Pharmacol. 76: 547–552, 1998.

22. Hackney AC. Characterization of the prolactin response to prolonged endurance exercise. Acta Kinesiologiae (University of Tartu). 13: 31–38, 2008.
23. Ansley L, G Marvin, A Sharma, MJ Kendall, DA Jones & MW Bridge. The effect of head cooling on endurance and neuroendocrine responses to exercise in warm conditions. Physiol Res. 57(6): 863–872, 2008.
24. Hackney AC, RJ Ness & A Schreiber. Effects of endurance exercise on nocturnal hormone concentrations in males. Chronobiol Int. 6(4): 341–346, 1989.
25. Hackney AC, MC Premo & RG McMurray. Influence of aerobic versus anaerobic exercise on the relationship between reproductive hormones in men. J Sports Sci. 13(4): 305–311, 1995.
26. Hackney AC, RL Sharp, WS Runyan & RJ Ness. Relationship of resting prolactin and testosterone changes in males during intensive training. British J Sports Med. 23(3): 194, 1989.
27. Wheeler GD, SR Wall, AN Belcastro & DC Cumming. Reduced serum testosterone and prolactin levels in male distance runners. JAMA. 252(4): 514–516, 1984.
28. Hackney AC, RL Sharp, W Runyan, Y Kim & RJ Ness. Effects of intensive training on the prolactin response to submaximal exercise in males. J Iowa Acad Sci. 96(2): 52–53, 1989.
29. Boyden TW, RW Pamenter, D Grosso, P Stanforth, T Rotkis & JH Wilmore. Prolactin responses, menstrual cycles, and body composition of women runners. J Clin Endocrinol Metab. 54(4): 711–714, 1982.
30. Hackney AC, WE Sinning & BC Bruot. Hypothalamic-pituitary-testicular axis function in endurance trained males. Int J Sports Med. 11: 298–303, 1990.
31. Hackney AC & JD Dobridge. Thyroid hormones and the interrelationship of cortisol and prolactin: influence of prolonged, exhaustive exercise. Pol J Endocrinol. 60(4): 252–257, 2009.
32. Ortega E. Neuroendocrine mediators in the modulation of phagocytosis by exercise: physiological implications. Exercise Immunol Rev. 9: 70–93, 2003.
33. Joyner M & EF Coyle. Endurance exercise performance: the physiology of champions. J Physiol. 586: 35–44, 2008.

Chapter 4
Exercise, Training, and the Hypothalamic–Pituitary–Gonadal Axis in Men

Michael Zitzmann

Introduction: An Association of the Gonadal Axis to Sports in Men?

There are numerous reports on the effects of physical exercise on testosterone levels and vice versa. Many of them lack control groups, have very low numbers of participants, or combine different effectors on hormone levels. Moreover, a distinction has to be made between physical exercises requiring endurance and those training strength.

Nevertheless, correlations between testosterone levels and various aspects of human behaviour and men's physical abilities have been widely examined. In this chapter, with a focus on controlled studies, interactions of androgens with physical and/or psychological phenomena and their applicability for individual purposes in sports are investigated.

An often neglected prerequisite in measuring testosterone levels in athletes is the consideration of the variance of secretion rates of this hormone as there exists a strong diurnal and also a measurable seasonal variation.

Testosterone levels and their bioavailable fractions are affected by weight, age, and diet. They are changed by different kinds of stress which may appear as physical stress (i.e., endurance training, sleep deprivation in extreme sports, changes of air pressure in altitude training) or mental stress (in relation to sport events and training). Pituitary reactivity to decreasing hormone levels seems too blunted in these situations.

Endurance Training and Physical Stress

Endurance training can have a prolonged effect on androgen levels. Most studies observed athletes during training and competition, giving the impression of generally lowered androgen levels, but lack the comparison with a control group.

M. Zitzmann (✉)
Centre for Reproductive Medicine and Andrology/Clinical Andrology,
University Clinics Müenster, Müenster, Germany
e-mail: michael.zitzmann@ukmuenster.de

E. Ghigo et al. (eds.), *Hormone Use and Abuse by Athletes*, Endocrine Updates 29,
DOI 10.1007/978-1-4419-7014-5_4, © Springer Science+Business Media, LLC 2011

A controlled study examining the effects of endurance training on the hypothalamic–pituitary–testicular axis in males involved 53 men undergoing endurance training for at least 5 years and a control group of 35 age-matched, sedentary men. Baseline serum testosterone levels of the exercising men were significantly lower than in the control group. Differences in gonadotropins were not seen. Normal regulation would require LH levels to rise with falling testosterone levels as these have a positive feedback on pituitary gonadotropin release. A suppression in the regulatory axis could explain this finding [1]. In a controlled exercise setting (which involved marathon athletes vs. sedentary men who performed defined running tests to reach fixed rates of their maximal heart rate), testosterone levels increased (being assessed immediately afterwards) in all men and the negative feedback of increasing testosterone levels on LH secretion could be described in both groups. The positive feedback of low testosterone levels was apparently insufficient in exercising men [2]. These results are similar to those of other studies with a controlled design [3, 4]. Mild prolonged physical exercise did not have major effects on testosterone levels in young type 1 diabetics versus an age-matched control group [5]. It has to be stressed that testosterone levels always stayed within the lower normal range.

That training and competition in physical endurance also means exposure to a physically and mentally stressful situation is shown by a controlled setting observing male participants of a 1-day ultramarathon (110 km). Testosterone levels were markedly decreased during the competition, and LH levels similar to above results did not change. In addition, cortisol levels as a endocrine marker for physical or mental stress exposure (see "mental stress") were elevated in runners in comparison to controls with high significance [6]. The effects of a 1,100 km run over 20 days were similar [7]. (For further results on stress and overtraining see [8–10].)

Hence, endurance training can be seen as a factor of exposure to physical stress. It has been demonstrated in a controlled study that the reactivity patterns of mental/psychological and physical stress responsivity of the hypothalamic–pituitary–adrenal axis are the same in a specific individual. Differential reactivity is rather seen between so-called high and low responders. Each group has a specific endocrine reactivity pattern concerning the hypothalamic–pituitary–adrenal axis [11].

Thus, the lowering effect of endurance training on testosterone levels might as well be seen as a matter of physical stress, being part of a general response pattern to stress in an individual. As described below, mental stress has a negative impact on testosterone secretion. In settings combining the two aspects of stress, testosterone levels can drop to clearly hypogonadal levels: a 5-day military training with physical activity during day and night, with almost no food or sleep found a marked decrease not only in testosterone but also in LH and FSH [12]. This was later confirmed by a similar study [13].

It seems that the decrease of testosterone levels under the stressful situations of endurance sport is not sufficiently answered by the pituitary. There is no adequate rise in LH levels, which seem to be unaltered or even show a tendency to decrease with the growing amount of stress impact.

Nevertheless, age-dependent effects seem to exist in this regard and the ratio of androgen to estradiol is shifted by physical activity to a more favourable pattern (higher androgen and lower estradiol levels) in older men compared to younger men performing regular mild physical activity [14].

Strength Training

Muscle mass and strength are often described to be significantly associated with testosterone levels, at least in males. This applies to elder men ($n = 121$) as well as to adolescents ($n = 87$) [15, 16].

Strength training can have an acute effect on endocrine functions. Immediate and 5 min postexercise measurement showed an increase in testosterone levels both in men and women [17]. This acute hormone response was confirmed and described to be markedly stronger in young men compared to old in a study involving ten men with mean age of 26.5 years and ten men with mean age of 70.0 years [18]. A longer lasting effect was measurable in eight young males performing 1-day intensive strength training: testosterone levels were elevated 24 h posttraining [19]. A similar result was seen in an equivalent setting involving 15 untrained males [20].

As muscle mass increases with strength training [21] and is correlated with testosterone levels (see above), it could be expected that testosterone levels also show a longer increase in persons constantly involved in strength training. A long-term training period of 12 weeks involving younger (mean 23 years) and older men (mean 63 years) showed no significant results concerning testosterone levels before or immediately after exercise [22]. Experienced weight lifters compared to beginners showed similar basal levels of testosterone but were able to evoke a stronger testosterone response during training [19]. Basal testosterone levels in trained weight lifters ($n = 11$) were not altered, nor did an increase in the daily training volume change these levels [23]. Short-term sprints can be seen as strength outburst and are comparable to strength training in general rather than endurance training: sprint training increases plasma testosterone concentrations in response to sprint exercise in adolescent boys. It has been speculated that plasma adrenaline and plasma lactate concentrations facilitate this physiological phenomenon [24].

Concerning moderate strength training, there seems to be no long-term effect on testosterone levels, though hormone levels are increased shortly after exercise. Overtraining as physical stress factor may decrease androgen levels.

Mental Stress of Sports

The release of cortisol by activation of the hypothalamic–pituitary–adrenal axis as a reaction to mental stress is well documented [11]. Stress responses by the hypothalamic–pituitary–gonadal axis are constantly found as well. This applies not only to physical stress but also to psychologically disturbing events. A sports event and also training for such can be seen as extremely mentally stressful.

In younger persons, physical stress but not mental stress seems to be able to exert a stimulatory role on the hypothalamic–pituitary–gonadal axis as well as the adrenal pathway [25]. However, this is obviously quite different in adult athletes.

Anticipatory stress was measured in 50 males before a 1-day experimental stress event (participation in stressfull clinical research protocol). Cortisol levels rose significantly, while both testosterone and LH secretion were decreased [26]. Psychological stress markers as measured by scales for anxiety, hostility, and depression were correlated with serum levels of testosterone in a group of males aged 30–55 years. Those classified as highly stressed had significantly lower testosterone levels than their counterparts [27]. A cross-sectional study involving 439 males all aged 51 years showed those with low levels of testosterone (adjusted for body mass index) to exhibit a cluster of psychosocial stress indicators [28]. The effect of stress release on testosterone levels was assessed in a study with volunteers assigned either to a group practising transcendental meditation or to a control group. The group learning to relax and to cope with stress had significantly decreasing levels of cortisol and significantly rising levels of serum testosterone [29]. The same effect was seen in 36 police inspectors threatened by unemployment and reorganisation. After the situation had changed for the better 3 years later, testosterone levels had clearly risen [30].

Hence, stressful events can clearly decrease serum testosterone levels, withdrawal from the situation is able to restore androgen levels. The response at the pituitary level is seen controversially. Some studies see LH secretion being decreased as well; others do not see any change. In summary, it remains unclear whether the drop of testosterone levels in mental stress exposure by sports is caused by decreased LH secretion or if an adequate response at the pituitary level is not given. Regarding the effects of physical stress of different degrees, probably the regulation of the pituitary–gonadal axis is suppressed according to the greater amount of impact. The first response, however, would be a decrease in testosterone levels with no appropriate reaction of the already suppressed LH secretion. If stress gets stronger, the LH levels already relatively low (in relation to low testosterone levels) drop below baseline values and are found to be absolutely decreased as well.

Conclusion

Testosterone secretion seems to be influenced not only by conditions which are partly controlled or initiated by the hormone itself, but also by circumstances beyond hormonal or individual control. One cannot estimate a person's testosterone level by the behaviour or physical appearance, as long as the individual is not in a hypogonadal state. This is rarely achieved by physical overtraining. Researching extragonadal actions of testosterone will yield restricted but valuable information on definite dimensions of male life and physical performance, not being immediately applicable to individual athletes.

References

1. Hackney AC, Sinning WE, Bruot BC. Hypothalamic-pituitary-testicular axis function endurance-trained males. Int J Sports Med. 1990; 11: 298–303.
2. Duclos M, Corcuff JB, Rashedi M, Fougere V, Manier G. Does functional alteration of the gonadotropic axis occur in endurance trained athletes during and after exercise? A preliminary study. Eur J Appl Physiol. 1996; 73: 427–433.
3. De Souza MJ, Arce JC, Pescatello LS, Scherzer HS, Luciano AA. Gonadal hormones and semen quality in male runners. A volume threshold effect of endurance training. Int J Sports Med. 1994; 15: 383–391.
4. Wheeler GD, Wall SR, Belcastro AN, Cumming DC. Reduced serum testosterone and prolactin levels in male distance runners. JAMA. 1984; 27: 514–516.
5. Berchtold P, Berger M, Cuppers HJ, Herrmann J, Nieschlag E, Rudorff K, Zimmermann H, Kruskemper HL. Non-glucoregulatory hormones (T4, T3, rT3, TSH, testosterone) during physical exercise in juvenile type diabetics. Horm Metab Res. 1978; 10: 269–273.
6. Fournier PE, Stalder J, Mermillod B, Chantraine A. Effects of a 110 kilometers ultra-marathon race on plasma hormone levels. Int J Sports Med. 1997; 18: 252–256.
7. Schuermeyer T, Jung K, Nieschlag E. The effect of an 1100 km run on testicular, adrenal and thyroid hormones. Int J Androl. 1984; 7: 276–282.
8. Chicharro JL, Lopez-Mojares LM, Lucia A, Perez M, Alvarez J, Labanda P, Calvo F, Vaquero AF. Overtraining parameters in special military units. Aviat Space Environ Med 1998; 69: 562–568.
9. Marinelli M, Roi GS, Giacometti M, Bonini P, Banfi G. Cortisol, testosterone, and free testosterone in athletes performing a marathon at 4,000 m altitude. Horm Res. 1994; 41: 225–229.
10. Vervoorn C, Quist AM, Vermulst LJ, Erich WB, de Vries WR, Thijssen JH. The behaviour of the plasma free testosterone/cortisol ratio during a season of elite rowing training. Int J Sports Med. 1991; 12: 257–263.
11. Singh A, Petrides JS, Gold PW, Chrousos GP, Deuster PA. Differential hypothalamic-pituitary-adrenal axis reactivity to psychological and physical stress. J Clin Endocrinol Metab. 1999; 84: 1944–1948.
12. Opstad PK. The hypothalamo-pituitary regulation of androgen secretion in young men after prolonged physical stress combined with energy and sleep deprivation. Acta Endocrinol (Copenh). 1992; 127: 231–236.
13. Bernton E, Hoover D, Galloway R, Popp K. Adaptation to chronic stress in military trainees. Adrenal androgens, testosterone, glucocorticoids, IGF-1, and immune function. Ann N Y Acad Sci. 1995; 29: 217–231.
14. Slowinska-Lisowska M, Jozkow P, Medras M. Associations between physical activity and the androgenic/estrogenic status of men. Physiol Res. 2010 Apr 20. [Epub ahead of print].
15. Baumgartner RN, Waters DL, Gallagher D, Morley JE, Garry PJ. Predictors of skeletal muscle mass in elderly men and women. Mech Ageing Dev. 1999; 107: 123–136.
16. Ramos E, Frontera WR, Llopart A, Feliciano D. Muscle strength and hormonal levels in adolescents: gender related differences. Int J Sports Med. 1998; 19: 526–531.
17. Kraemer WJ, Staron RS, Hagerman FC, Hikida RS, Fry AC, Gordon SE, Nindl BC, Gothshalk LA, Volek JS, Marx JO, Newton RU, Hakkinen K. The effects of short-term resistance training on endocrine function in men and women. Eur J Appl Physiol. 1998; 78: 69–76.
18. Hakkinen K, Pakarinen A, Newton RU, Kraemer WJ. Acute hormone responses to heavy resistance lower and upper extremity exercise in young versus old men. Eur J Appl Physiol. 1998; 77: 312–319.
19. Kraemer RR, Kilgore JL, Kraemer GR, Castracane VD. Growth hormone, IGF-I, and testosterone responses to resistive exercise. Med Sci Sports Exerc. 1992; 24: 1346–1352.
20. Jurimae T, Karelson K, Smirnova T, Viru A. The effect of a single-circuit weight-training session on the blood biochemistry of untrained university students. Eur J Appl Physiol. 1990; 61: 344–348.

21. Bhasin S, Storer TW, Berman N, Callegari C, Clevenger B, Phillips J, Bunnell TJ, Tricker R, Shirazi A, Casaburi R. The effects of supraphysiologic doses of testosterone on muscle size and strength in normal men. N Engl J Med. 1996; 335: 1–7.
22. Craig BW, Brown R, Everhart J. Effects of progressive resistance training on growth hormone and testosterone levels in young and elderly subjects. Mech Ageing Dev. 1989; 49: 159–169.
23. Fry AC, Kraemer WJ, Ramsey LT. Pituitary-adrenal-gonadal responses to high-intensity resistance exercise overtraining. J Appl Physiol. 1998; 85: 2352–2359.
24. Derbré F, Vincent S, Maitel B, Jacob C, Delamarche P, Delamarche A, Zouhal H. Androgen responses to sprint exercise in young men. Int J Sports Med. 2010; 31: 291–297.
25. Budde H, Pietrassyk-Kendziorra S, Bohm S, Voelcker-Rehage C. Hormonal responses to physical and cognitive stress in a school setting. Neurosci Lett. 2010; 474: 131–134.
26. Schulz P, Walker JP, Peyrin L, Soulier V, Curtin F, Steimer T. Lower sex hormones in men during anticipatory stress. Neuroreport. 1996; 25; 3101–3104.
27. Francis KT. The relationship between high and low trait psychological stress, serum testosterone, and serum cortisol. Experientia. 1981; 37(12): 1296–1297.
28. Nilsson PM, Moller L, Solstad K. Adverse effects of psychosocial stress on gonadal function and insulin levels in middle-aged males. J Intern Med. 1995; 237: 479–486.
29. MacLean CR, Walton KG, Wenneberg SR, Levitsky DK, Mandarino JP, Waziri R, Hillis SL, Schneider RH. Effects of the transcendental meditation program on adaptive mechanisms: changes in hormone levels and responses to stress after 4 months of practice. Psychoneuroendocrinology. 1997; 22: 277–295.
30. Grossi G, Theorell T, Jurisoo M, Setterlind S. Psychophysiological correlates of organizational change and threat of unemployment among police inspectors. Integr Physiol Behav Sci. 1999; 34: 30–42.

Chapter 5
Exercise and the Reproductive System in Women

Anne B. Loucks

Introduction

Unless dietary intake is raised to compensate for the energy cost of exercise, investigators will misinterpret effects of energy deficiency as effects of exercise [1]. The first investigator of the female reproductive system to do so was Hans Selye, who reported in 1939 that "the ovaries undergo atrophy and more or less permanent anestrus ensues" when young female rats were forced to exercise for prolonged periods [2]. Selye observed a *General Adaptation Syndrome* also involving hypertrophy of the adrenal glands, cessation of growth and lactation, shrinkage of the liver, loss of muscular tone, a fall in body temperature, and the disappearance of adipose tissue [3]. These and other apparent effects of prolonged exercise and other nocuous agents occurred dramatically during an initial 2-day alarm stage, then slowly during a prolonged resistant stage before ending in a rapidly fatal exhaustion stage. Selye noticed that withholding food shortened the resistant stage, during which the animal "learns to perform adaptive functions more economically and with less dependence on the caloric energy derived from food" [4]. He hypothesized that "adaptation of the organism is dependent upon a special hitherto unrecognized type of energy," which he called *adaptation energy*, that was slowly consumed during the resistant stage. Yet it did not occur to Selye that adaptation energy was the energy stored in adipose tissue or that his rats were starving, because the role of adipose tissue in energy metabolism was unknown at the time [5]. He did not check whether increasing dietary intake would prevent the General Adaptation Syndrome, and concluded that it must be caused by a biological phenomenon that he had discovered for the first time. He called this phenomenon *stress*. Only in recent years have investigators learned that the various features of the General Adaptation Syndrome can be prevented by increasing dietary intake and other means for supplementing the organism's supply of energy, particularly carbohydrate (CHO) [6].

A.B. Loucks (✉)
Department of Biological Sciences, Ohio University, Athens, OH, USA
e-mail: loucks@ohio.edu

E. Ghigo et al. (eds.), *Hormone Use and Abuse by Athletes*, Endocrine Updates 29, DOI 10.1007/978-1-4419-7014-5_5, © Springer Science+Business Media, LLC 2011

Effects of Exercise Training on LH Pulsatility in Women

LH Pulsatility

Ovarian function depends on the pulsatile secretion of luteinizing hormone (LH) by the pituitary gland. Athletes with suppressed luteal function secrete a reduced number of LH pulses at regular intervals, and those with functional hypothalamic amenorrhea (FHA) secrete even fewer pulses at irregular intervals [7]. Athletes also display diverse metabolic abnormalities characteristic of energy deficiency proportional to the severity of their reproductive disorders [8].

Independent Effects of Exercise Training on LH Pulsatility

In imitation of Selye, we abruptly imposed a high volume of intense exercise on healthy, young, regularly menstruating, untrained women of normal body composition [9]. For 4 days, each woman walked on a motorized treadmill at 70% of her aerobic capacity until she had expended 30 kilocalories per kilogram of fat-free mass each day (kcal/kgFFM/day), which was similar to the energy cost of running a half-marathon each day.

Unlike Selye, we administered this exercise regimen twice, with and without dietary supplementation for the energy cost of the exercise. We also studied a second group of similar women, who remained sedentary, with and without dietary restriction in the same amount as the increased energy expenditure of the exercising group. Defining energy availability operationally as dietary energy intake minus exercise energy expenditure, we manipulated diets to administer the same balanced and low energy availabilities of 45 and 10 kcal/kgFFM/day to both groups.

We found that low energy availability suppressed LH pulse frequency and that exercise had no suppressive effect on LH pulsatility beyond the impact of its energy cost on energy availability. Later experiments on female monkeys induced amenorrhea by increasing the volume of exercise training without increasing dietary energy intake [10] and then restored ovulation by increasing dietary energy intake without moderating the exercise regimen [11]. We were surprised to notice, however, that the disruption of LH pulsatility by low energy availability in our exercising women was smaller than that in our dietarily restricted women.

Effects of Gynecological Age (Years Since Menarche)

Subsequently, we administered the same energy availabilities to similar older adolescent women 5–8 years of gynecological age (~20 years of calendar age) and young adult women 14–18 years of gynecological age (~29 years of calendar age), and found that the sensitivity of LH pulsatility to low energy availability disappeared between 8 and 14 years of gynecological age [12]. This was consistent with the much higher prevalence of amenorrhea in runners <15 years of gynecological age than in older runners [13], and with the declining prevalence of menstrual disorders during adolescence [14] as fertility increases [15].

Dose–Response Effects of Energy Availability

To investigate the dose–response relationship between energy availability and LH pulsatility in exercising women [16], we administered balanced and one of three low energy availabilities (45 and either 10, 20, or 30 kcal/kgFFM/day) to healthy, habitually sedentary, regularly menstruating, older adolescent women for 5 days. LH pulsatility was disrupted only below 30 kcal/kgFFM/day. This was consistent with many studies of amenorrheic runners, all of which indicated energy availabilities <30 kcal/kgFFM/day [17], and with the only prospective study of the refeeding of amenorrheic athletes, in which menstrual cycles were restored in runners by increasing energy availability from 25 to 31 kcal/kgFFM/day [18].

Associated Effects on Metabolic Hormones and Substrates

Independent Effects of Exercise Training

While investigating LH pulsatility [9], we found that several metabolic substrates and hormones were also disrupted by low energy availability and not by exercise training, and their disruptions were also smaller in exercising women than in dietarily restricted women. At first, we suspected that the two groups of women were somehow different from one another, but we found nothing explanatory in a wide range of historical, anthropometric, and physiological data.

So we checked whether the exercising women had more CHO available, even though their energy availability had been the same as the sedentary women. Defining CHO availability observationally as dietary CHO intake minus CHO oxidation during exercise, we found that the exercising women had oxidized much less CHO during the low energy availability treatment than during the balanced energy availability treatment. As a result, their CHO availability was 70% higher than that of the dietarily restricted women during the low energy availability treatment, so that the CHO availability of the dietarily restricted women was less and that of the exercising women was more than the brain glucose requirement of 90 g/day.

Effects of Gynecological Age

Although low energy availability did not disrupt LH pulsatility in exercising adults, it did disrupt their metabolic substrates and hormones as much or more than those of the exercising adolescents [12]. This suggested three possible explanations for the insensitivity of LH pulsatility to low energy availability in the adults. First, central nervous system sensitivity to signals of energy deficiency may decline during adolescence. Second, competition from peripheral tissues against the brain for metabolic fuels may decline with growth rate. Third, adults may mobilize more fatty acids from adipose tissue under energy-deficient conditions.

Dose–Response Effects of Energy Availability

As energy availability was reduced [16], metabolic substrates and hormones displayed distinctive dose–response relationships. Insulin declined linearly, but T_3 and IGF-I declined and GH rose abruptly as energy availability declined from 30 to 20 kcal/kgFFM/day. This hepatic GH resistance reflected the modulation of hepatic sensitivity to GH by T_3, the level of which depends on CHO availability. Cortisol rose exponentially. Leptin was already substantially suppressed at 30 kcal/kgFFM/day, and declined only a little more as energy availability was further reduced, so that its dose–response relationship was very different from that of LH pulsatility. These and other glucoregulatory responses maintained plasma glucose levels down to 30 kcal/kgFFM/day with only a slight increase in β-hydroxybutyrate (i.e., lipolysis and β-oxidation of fatty acids), but more extreme responses were unable to prevent plasma glucose from declining and an exponential increase in β-hydroxybutyrate below that threshold.

The Dose–Response Effects of Energy Availability on Bone Turnover

Because athletes with FHA frequently display low bone mineral densities, we also assessed the dose–response effects of energy availability on markers of bone turnover in the same women in whom we had determined other dose–response relationships [19]. As expected, bone resorption increased only when energy availability was reduced sufficiently to suppress estradiol, but bone formation was suppressed at much higher energy availabilities. The rate of synthesis of type I collagen in the bone protein matrix declined linearly with energy availability, like insulin, which regulates collagen synthesis. Meanwhile, the mineralization of that protein matrix declined abruptly between 30 and 20 kcal/kgFFM/day, like T_3 and IGF-I, which regulate the synthesis of osteocalcin, the protein that binds calcium to type I bone collagen.

Comparison of Experimental Results to the Female Athlete Triad

The revised American College of Sports Medicine (ACSM) position stand on the Female Athlete Triad clarifies that the Triad refers specifically and only to the physiological mechanisms by which low energy availability disrupts reproductive function and impairs bone mineral density [20]. The Triad spans wide spectrums of energy availability, menstrual function, and bone mineral density between health and disease, and it is not restricted to eating disorders, amenorrhea, and osteoporosis at the pathological ends of those spectrums. Although reproductive disorders in the Triad are functional in nature, they still require prompt intervention to prevent potentially irreversible losses of bone mineral and increased risks of stress fractures in the near term and osteoporotic fractures later in life. Because restoring regular menstrual cycles with birth control pills does not correct the chronic under-nutrition that causes the Triad, the first aim of treatment for the Triad is to increase energy availability.

References

1. Braun B, Brooks GA. Critical importance of controlling energy status to understand the effects of "exercise" on metabolism. Exerc Sport Sci Rev 2008; 36:2–4.
2. Selye H. The effect of adaptation to various damaging agents on the female sex organs in the rat. Endocrinology 1939; 25:615–624.
3. Selye H. A syndrome produced by diverse nocuous agents. Nature 1936; 138:32.
4. Selye H. Adaptation energy. Nature 1938; 141:926.
5. Wertheimer H. Introduction – a perspective. In: Renold A, Cahill G Jr, eds. Handbook of Physiology Section 5: Adipose Tissue. Washington: American Physiological Society 1965; 5–11.
6. Loucks A. Is stress measured in joules? Military Psychol 2009; 21:S101–S107.
7. Loucks AB, Mortola JF, Girton L, Yen SSC. Alterations in the hypothalamic-pituitary-ovarian and the hypothalamic-pituitary-adrenal axes in athletic women. J Clin Endocrinol Metab 1989; 68:402–411.
8. Laughlin GA, Yen SSC. Nutritional and endocrine-metabolic aberrations in amenorrheic athletes. J Clin Endocrinol Metab 1996; 81:4301–4309.
9. Loucks AB, Verdun M, Heath EM. Low energy availability, not stress of exercise, alters LH pulsatility in exercising women. J Appl Physiol 1998; 84:37–46.
10. Williams NI, Caston-Balderrama AL, Helmreich DL, Parfitt DB, Nosbisch C, Cameron JL. Longitudinal changes in reproductive hormones and menstrual cyclicity in cynomolgus monkeys during strenuous exercise training: abrupt transition to exercise-induced amenorrhea. Endocrinology 2001; 142:2381–2389.
11. Williams NI, Helmreich DL, Parfitt DB, Caston-Balderrama AL, Cameron JL. Evidence for a causal role of low energy availability in the induction of menstrual cycle disturbances during strenuous exercise training. J Clin Endocrinol Metab 2001; 86:5184–5193.
12. Loucks AB. The response of luteinizing hormone pulsatility to five days of low energy availability disappears by 14 years of gynecological age. J Clin Endocrinol Metab 2006; 91:3158–3164.
13. Baker ER, Mathur RS, Kirk RF, Williamson HO. Female runners and secondary amenorrhea: correlation with age, parity, mileage, and plasma hormonal and sex-hormone-binding globulin concentrations. Fertil Steril 1981; 36:183–187.

14. Vollman RF. The menstrual cycle. In: Friedman EA, ed. Major Problems in Obstetrics and Gynecology, Vol 7. Philadelphia: W.B. Saunders 1977:193.
15. Ellison PT. Advances in human reproductive ecology. Annu Rev Anthropol 1994; 23:255–275.
16. Loucks AB, Thuma JR. Luteinizing hormone pulsatility is disrupted at a threshold of energy availability in regularly menstruating women. J Clin Endocrinol Metab 2003; 88:297–311.
17. Loucks AB. Low energy availability in the marathon and other endurance sports. Sports Med 2007; 37:348–52.
18. Kopp-Woodroffe SA, Manore MM, Dueck CA, Skinner JS, Matt KS. Energy and nutrient status of amenorrheic athletes participating in a diet and exercise training intervention program. Int J Sport Nutr 1999; 9:70–88.
19. Ihle R, Loucks AB. Dose-response relationships between energy availability and bone turn-over in young exercising women. J Bone Miner Res 2004; 19:1231–1240.
20. Nattiv A, Loucks AB, Manore MM, Sundgot-Borgen J, Warren MP. American College of Sports Medicine Position Stand: The female athlete triad. Med Sci Sports Exerc 2007; 39:1867–1882.

Chapter 6
Physical Exercise, Sports, and Diabetes

Pierpaolo de Feo

Introduction

Today, more than 1.1 billion adults are overweight, and 312 billion of them are obese; the people with diabetes is projected to increase from 171 to 366 million in 2030 [1]. The increase in the prevalence of obesity and the incidence of type 2 diabetes among children is predictive of alarming consequences [1, 2].

We should apply all our efforts to use physical activity to prevent and cure these diseases. In this regard, a crucial role is played by the effects of physical inactivity and of exercise on mitochondrial biogenesis in skeletal muscle [3]. Skeletal muscle represents about 80–90% of all insulin-sensitive tissues and accounts for about 50% of basal metabolic rate [4]. Epidemiological studies have shown a significant inverse relationship between the level of physical fitness and the prevalence of metabolic syndrome either in adults [5] or in children [6]. In rats, genetic selection for low maximal oxygen transport capacity (VO_{2max}), an objective measure of physical fitness, leads to the typical features of the metabolic syndrome [7]. Additionally, in humans, low values of VO_{2max} and of mitochondrial functional capacity are strictly related with reduced insulin sensitivity [8]. Several studies have demonstrated mitochondrial dysfunction in subjects with insulin resistance, obesity, and/or type 2 diabetes [8]. There are also several studies demonstrating that regular aerobic exercise can increase VO_{2max} and partially reverse mitochondrial dysfunction by stimulating mitochondrial biogenesis and augmenting mitochondrial oxidative capacity [9, 10]. The effectiveness of a training program to treat diabetes is a function of age of subjects and of type, frequency, intensity, and duration of exercise.

P. de Feo (✉)
Department of Internal Medicine, C.U.R.I.A.MO (Centro Universitario Ricerca Interdipartimentale Attività Motoria), University of Perugia, Perugia, Italy
e-mail: pierpaolodefeo@gmail.com

E. Ghigo et al. (eds.), *Hormone Use and Abuse by Athletes*, Endocrine Updates 29,
DOI 10.1007/978-1-4419-7014-5_6, © Springer Science+Business Media, LLC 2011

Aging, Physical Activity, and Type 2 Diabetes Mellitus

Aging is associated with reduced muscle oxidative capacity [11, 12], probably due to a reduction of the content and/or mitochondrial function [13]. Low oxidative capacity of skeletal muscle is also associated with insulin resistance [14] and type 2 diabetes mellitus [15, 16]. In 2008, Rönn et al. published a work based on biopsies of vast lateral muscle in nondiabetic young or elderly twins, which shows that in older people there is a reduced expression of mRNAm of gene COX7A1 [17]. The gene COX7A1 is a component of the respiratory chain whose reduced expression has been demonstrated in type 2 diabetes mellitus [15]. In the study of Rönn et al., the expression of COX7A1 is correlated with VO_{2max} (maximum capacity to carry oxygen), the ability to transport glucose, and the expression of PGC-1α, a key activator of mitochondrial biogenesis. In people with type 2 diabetes, it has already been demonstrated that either the expression of PGC-1α [15], the VO_{2max}, or the ability to transport glucose is reduced compared with nondiabetic controls [18]. It has also been shown that regular exercise increases the oxidative capacity of skeletal muscle [19–21]. It has been shown that aerobic training of long duration in elderly men and women increases mitochondrial protein content [22] and volume [23]. More recently, it has been confirmed that in healthy old subjects, a 12-week aerobic exercise increases the mitochondrial DNA content and activity [24]. These data show that biogenesis and mitochondrial function maintain a good response to exercise even in the elderly, in good health. Recent studies show that the mitochondria of skeletal muscle of subjects with type 2 diabetes is smaller and less efficient than those of controls without diabetes [8]. Exercise improves insulin sensitivity, VO_{2max}, the number of mitochondria, cardiolipin content, and mitochondrial oxidative enzymes in patients with type 2 diabetes mellitus with a mean age of 44 ± 3 years [25]. There are no studies in older people with DM2. However, considering that the beneficial effects of physical activity are independent of age in DM2 [26], we can reasonably assume that adaptive responses in mitochondrial content and activity to exercise also occur in elderly DM2 subjects.

Type, Frequency, Intensity, and Duration of Exercise

A meta-analysis of the few controlled studies that evaluated the effects of interventions based on structured physical activity in type 2 diabetes shows an improvement of around 0.6–0.7% in average HBA1c [26, 27]. Most of these studies assessed the type of aerobic activity, but some data suggest that muscle strength training may have similar benefits [28–31]. It is likely that this result is achieved through different molecular mechanisms with the two types of exercise and that they can be synergistic [32]. For this reason, the American Diabetes Association (ADA) recommends at least 150 min/week of moderate aerobic physical activity that should be combined with three weekly sessions of resistance exercise to increase muscle strength [33].

In DM2 subjects, there is a strict positive relationship between the amount of energy expenditure due to exercise and the improvements of several metabolic and anthropometric parameters [34]. Thus, regarding the amount of physical activity, it is recommended to start the training program with reasonable targets, well-matched with time availability and self-esteem of patients [35]. Once subjects experience the beneficial effects of the life-style change, it is important to augment the amount of energy expenditure achievable through physical activity in order to maximize the benefits. It has been estimated that most of the beneficial effects in terms of improvement in metabolic and anthropometric parameters, reduction of cardiovascular risk, and drug consumption are achieved with 35 (metabolic equivalent) METs/h/week [34].

The intensity of exercise should be in the moderate range (3–6 MET) for several reasons. Usually, DM2 subjects are not familiar with high-intensity workouts and could easily drop out; the risk of acute cardiovascular events increases with the intensity of exercise; moderate intensity exercise can be sustained for prolonged time. A training planned on moderate intensity/long distances favors lipid consumption [36] and increases insulin sensitivity up to 14 days after the end of the last exercise session [37].

Exercise Counseling

Despite the evidence about the benefits of exercise, many physicians do not spend time and effort to convince type 2 diabetic subjects to practice physical activity. There is the need for simple and reproducible strategies of counseling to motivate type 2 diabetic patients to exercise [38]. We and others have demonstrated that using an individual behavioral approach, it is possible for physicians to motivate the majority of type 2 diabetic subjects to practice regular long-term exercise [35, 38].

In a first counseling of at least 30 min, our intervention is to advise physical activity, followed by home calling after 1 month and by an ambulatory visit of about 15 min for every 3 months [35]. The counseling session is structured in seven points: (1) (motivation) the physician explains the beneficial effects of exercise as reported by the scientific literature for the general population and, specifically, for DM2 subjects, stressing those that are more appealing to individual patients; (2) (self-efficacy) the physician and the patient agree on an exercise program, which could be positively performed, characterized by increasing tasks; (3) (pleasure) the physician suggests at least two to three different types of physical activities, from among which the patient selects the ones which he or she considers more interesting or workable; (4) (support) the partner of the patient, when present, is invited to share with her/him the sessions of physical activity; (5) (comprehension) the physician listens to the patient to make sure that she/he really appreciates the advantages of the behavioral change; (6) (lack of impediments) the physician facilitates the patient to find a solution for potential obstacles to the regular practice of physical exercise; (7) (diary) the patient is asked to report daily, the type and amount of physical activity. On subsequent visits (once every 3 months), the diary is used to record the amount of physical activity reported and to encourage the self-efficacy of the patients. These visits are also used to promote the duration or the number of sessions of physical exercise, to solve the practical problems related to the physical activity of the patient, and to modify the treatment, if necessary. Using this structured behavioral approach, about 70% of type 2 diabetic patients achieved the goal of an energy expenditure through voluntary physical activity greater than 10 MET/h/week [35].

References

1. Hossain P, Kawar B et al. Obesity and diabetes in the developing world – a growing challenge. N Engl J Med 2007; 356: 213–215.
2. Maffeis C. Physical activity: an effective way to control weight in children? Nutr Metab Cardiovasc Dis 2007; 17: 394–408.
3. Hood DA, Salem A. Exercise-induced mitochondrial biogenesis in skeletal muscle. Nutr Metab Cardiovasc Dis 2007; 17: 332–337.
4. Baron AD, Brechtel G, Wallace P, Edelman SV. Rates and tissue sites on non-insulin- and insulin-mediated glucose uptake in humans. Am J Physiol 1988; 255: E769–E774.
5. Laaksonen DE et al. Low levels of leisure-time physical activity and cardiorespiratory fitness predict development of the metabolic syndrome. Diabetes Care 2002; 25: 1612–1618.
6. Brage S et al. European Youth Heart Study (EYHS). Features of the metabolic syndrome are associated with objectively measured physical activity and fitness in Danish children: the European Youth Heart Study (EYHS). Diabetes Care 2004; 27: 2141–2148.
7. Wisloff U, Najjar SM et al. Cardiovascular risk factors emerge after artificial selection for low aerobic capacity. Science 2005; 307: 418–420.
8. Kelley DE et al. Dysfunction of mitochondria in human skeletal muscle in type 2 diabetes. Diabetes 2002; 51: 2944–2950.
9. De Feo P, Stocchi V. Physical activity for the treatment and prevention of metabolic syndrome. Nutr Metab Cardiovasc Dis 2007; 17: 327–331.
10. Guescini M et al. Fine needle aspiration coupled with real-time PCR: a painless methodology to study adaptive functional changes in skeletal muscle. Nutr Metab Cardiovasc Dis 2007; 17: 383–393.
11. Cooper JM, Mann VM, Shapira AH. Analyses of mitochondrial respiratory chain function and mitochondrial DNA deletion in human skeletal muscle: effect of ageing. J Neurol Sci 1992; 98: 113–191.
12. Coggan AR, Spina RJ, Kings DS, Rogers MA, Brown M, Nemeth PM, Holloszy JO. Histochemical and enzymatic comparison of the gastrocnemius muscle of young and ederly men and women. J Gerontol 1992; 47: B71–B76.
13. Short KR, Bigelow ML, Kahl J et al. Decline in skeletal muscle mitochondrial function with aging in humans. Proc Natl Acad Sci USA 2005; 102: 5618–5623.
14. Simoneau JA, Colberg SR, Thaete FL, Kelley DE. Skeletal muscle glycolitic and oxidative enzyme capacities are determinants of insulin sensitivity and muscle composition in obese women. FASEB J 1995; 9: 273-278.
15. Mootha V, Lindgren CM, Eriksson KF et al. PGC-1alpha responsive genes involved in oxidative phosphorylation are co-ordinately downregulated in human diabetes. Nat Genet 2003; 34: 267–273.

16. Patti M, Butte A, Crunkhorn S et al. Coordinated reduction on genes of oxidative metabolism in humans with insulin resistance and diabetes: potential roles of PGC1 and NRF-1. Proc Natl Acad Sci USA 2003, 100: 8466–8471.
17. Rönn T, Poulsen P, Hansson O et al. Age influences DNA methylation and gene expression of COX7A1 in human skeletal muscle. Diabetologia 2008; 51: 1159–1168.
18. De Feo P, Di Loreto C, Ranchelli A et al. Physical inactivity is the main cause of the metabolic syndrome. In: Stocchi V, de Feo P, Hood DA (eds) Role of physical exercise in preventing disease and improving the quality of life. Milan: Springer 2007; 23–33.
19. Dohm GL, Huston RL, Askew EW, Fleshood HL. Effects of exercise, training, and diet on muscle citric acid cycle enzyme activity. Can J Biochem 1973; 51: 849–854.
20. Holloszy JO, Oscai LB, Dohn IJ, Molé PA. Mitochondrial citric acid cycle and related enzymes: adaptive response to exercise. Biochem Biophys Res Commun 1970; 40: 1368–1373.
21. Hoppeler H, Luthi P, Claassen H, Weibel ER, Howald H. The ultrastructure of the normal human skeletal muscle. A morphometric analysis on untrained men, women and well trained orienteers. Pfuegers Arch 1973; 344: 217–232.
22. Coggan AR, Spina RJ, Kings DS, Rogers MA, Brown M, Nemeth PM, Holloszy JO. Skeletal muscle adaptations to endurance training in 60- to 70-yr-old men and women. J Appl Physiol 1992; 72: 1780–1786.
23. Jubrias SA, Esselman PC, Price LB, Cress ME, Conley KE. Large energetic adaptations of ederly muscle to resistance and endurance training. J Appl Physiol 2001; 90: 1663–1670.
24. Menshikova EV, Ritov VB, Fairfull L, Ferrell RE, Kelley DE, Goodpaster BH. Effects of exercise on mitochondrial content and function in aging human skeletal muscle. J Gerontol A Biol Sci Med Sci 2006; 61: 534–540.
25. Toledo FGS, Menshikova EV, Ritov VB, Azuma K, Radikova Z, DeLany J, Kelley DE. Effects of physical activity and weight loss on skeletal muscle mitochondria and relationship with glucose control in type 2 diabetes. Diabetes 2007; 56: 2142–2147.
26. Boulé NG, Haddad E, Kenny GP, Wells GA, Sigal RJ. Effects of exercise on glycemic control and body mass in type 2 diabetes mellitus: a meta-analysis of controlled clinical trials. JAMA 2001; 286: 1218–1227.
27. Thomas DE, Elliott EJ, Naughton GA. Exercise for type 2 diabetes mellitus. Cochrane Database Syst Rev 2006; (3): CD002968.
28. Dunstan DW, Daly RM, Owen N, Jolley D, De Courten M, Shaw J, Zimmet P. High-intensity resistance training improves glycemic control in older patients with type 2 diabetes. Diabetes Care 2002; 25: 1729–1736.
29. Castaneda C, Layne JE, Munoz-Orians L, Gordon PL, Walsmith J, Foldvari M, Roubenoff R, Tucker KL, Nelson ME. A randomized controlled trial of resistance exercise training to improve glycemic control in older adults with type 2 diabetes. Diabetes Care 2002; 25: 2335–2341.
30. Balducci S, Leonetti F, Di Mario U, Fallucca F. Is a long-term aerobic plus resistance training program feasible for and effective on metabolic profiles in type 2 diabetic patients? Diabetes Care 2004; 27: 841–842.
31. Sigal RJ, Kenny GP, Boulé NG, Wells GA, Prud'homme D, Fortier M, Reid RD, Tulloch H, Coyle D, Phillips P, Jennings A, Jaffey J. Effects of aerobic training, resistance training, or both on glycemic control in type 2 diabetes: a randomized trial. Ann Intern Med. 2007; 147: 357–369.
32. Kraus WE, Levine BD. Exercise training for diabetes: the "strength" of the evidence. Ann Intern Med 2007; 147: 423–424.
33. Sigal RJ, Kenny GP, Wasserman DH, Castaneda-Sceppa C, White RD. Physical activity/ exercise and type 2 diabetes: a consensus statement from the American Diabetes Association. Diabetes Care 2006; 29: 1433–1438.
34. Di Loreto C, Fanelli C, Lucidi P, et al. Make your diabetic patients walk: long-term impact of different amounts of physical activity on type 2 diabetes. Diabetes Care 2005; 28: 1295–1302.

35. Di Loreto C, Fanelli C, Lucidi P et al. Validation of a counseling strategy to promote the adoption and the maintenance of physical activity by type 2 diabetic subjects. Diabetes Care 2003; 26: 404–408.
36. De Feo P, Di Loreto C, Lucidi P, Murdolo G, Parlanti N, De Cicco A, Piccioni F, Santeusanio F. Metabolic response to exercise. J Endocrinol Invest 2003; 26: 851–854.
37. Bajpeyi S, Tanner CJ, Slentz CA, Duscha BD, McCartney JS, Hickner RC, Kraus WE, Houmard JA. Effect of exercise intensity and volume on the persistence of insulin sensitivity during training cessation. J Appl Physiol 2009; 106: 1079–1085.
38. Kirk A, De Feo P. Strategies to enhance compliance to physical activity for patients with insulin resistance. Appl Physiol Nutr Metab 2007; 32: 549–556.

Chapter 7
Motor Performance and Muscle Mass as a Function of Hormonal Responses to Exercise

Marco A. Minetto, Andrea Benso, Ezio Ghigo, and Fabio Lanfranco

Neuro-Endocrine–Muscular Interactions in Response to Acute Exercise

In this section, we focus on the metabotropic actions exerted by (neuro)hormones and neurotransmitters on the nerve cells, known as motoneurons, which control the excitation of the muscle fibers. In the muscle, each fiber is activated by a single motoneuron, but each motoneuron innervates from tens to thousands of muscle fibers. The motor unit (one motor neuron and all the muscle fibers that its axon innervates) denotes the basic functional element of the central nervous system and muscle that produces movement. Its function is to transform synaptic input received by the motoneuron into mechanical output by the muscle [1]. As exemplified in Fig. 7.1, the synaptic input to motoneurons is ionotropic and metabotropic [2, 3]. Some of the ionotropic input is monosynaptic sensory input from the periphery, but most is represented by supra-spinal input which passes through various types of spinal interneurons. Ionotropic (voltage-regulated) actions on spinal motoneurons are triggered by excitatory and inhibitory postsynaptic potentials [3]. Metabotropic (neuromodulatory) actions involve synaptic or hormonal inputs acting in many cases via G-protein-coupled receptors embedded in the neuron membrane. Metabotropic descending input sets the excitability of the dendrites of the spinal motoneurons by triggering conductance changes on the motoneuron membranes and producing persistent inward currents [2]. The capacity of motoneuron dendrites to generate persistent inward currents (and their dependence on neuromodulatory inputs) implies that muscle force production (and modulation) largely results from the degree to which ionotropic inputs activate these excitable dendrites. The metabotropic drive that makes the motoneuron dendrites hyperexcitable, and that is likely to occur in "fight or flight" situations, should allow of the generation of very high forces for very modest input levels. A variety of neuromodulators (i.e., agents that trigger metabotropic actions)

M.A. Minetto (✉)
Division of Endocrinology and Metabolism, Department of Internal Medicine,
University of Turin, Turin, Italy
e-mail: marcominetto@libero.it

E. Ghigo et al. (eds.), *Hormone Use and Abuse by Athletes*, Endocrine Updates 29,
DOI 10.1007/978-1-4419-7014-5_7, © Springer Science+Business Media, LLC 2011

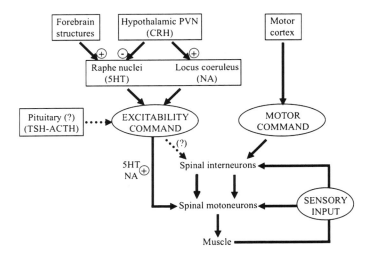

Fig. 7.1 Descending and sensory control of motoneurons during movement. *Right-side* connections show the motor command emanating from the motor cortex (and other regions of the central nervous system) and sensory inputs from the periphery, which converge on spinal interneurons, which exerts ionotropic actions on spinal motoneurons. *Left-side* connections show the excitability command arising from metabotropic (neuromodulatory) descending inputs, which control the excitability of spinal motoneurons via the actions of serotonin (5HT) and noradrenaline (NA). *Question marks* and *broken arrows* indicate possibilities under investigation. *PVN* paraventricular nuclei, *CRH* corticotrophin-releasing hormone, *TSH* thyroid-stimulating hormone, *ACTH* adrenocorticotropic hormone. Modified from Heckman et al. [2]

are known to act on spinal motoneurons, including the monoamines serotonin (5HT) and noradrenaline (NA) (which are produced, respectively, by neurons in the raphe nuclei and locus coeruleus of the brainstem), the neurotransmitters acetylcoline, glutamate, GABA (which also exert ionotropic actions), and, possibly, some pituitary hormones (thyroid-stimulating hormone and adrenocorticotropic hormone) [2].

The neuro-endocrine response to exercise may play a role in regulating the level of neuromodulatory input to motoneurons: in fact, it consists of a stereotyped response, called *stress response*, whose main components are the activations of the hypothalamic–pituitary–adrenal axis and the systemic sympathetic and adreno medullary systems [4]. The pituitary–adrenal excitation is controlled by the liberation of corticotrophin-releasing hormone (CRH), by the hypothalamic paraventricular nuclei, into the pituitary portal system of the median eminence. In addition to its action on the anterior pituitary, CRH is thought to function as a brain neurotransmitter to activate the brain noradrenergic nucleus, locus coeruleus [5]. This is supported by ultrastructural evidence for synaptic specializations between CRH-immunoreactive terminals and locus coeruleus dendrites [6]. Moreover, CRH administered into the locus coeruleus increased both the discharge rates of locus coeruleus neurons [7] and the noradrenaline release in locus coeruleus target regions [7]. CRH and noradrenergic neurons innervate and activate each other and are stimulated by the serotonergic and cholinergic systems. In addition, the serotonergic dorsal raphe nucleus is innervated by CRH neurons and expresses CRH receptors, suggesting that endogenous CRH impacts on this system [8]. Price et al. [9] and Waselus et al. [10] provided neurochemical and electrophysiological evidence that CRH has both direct and indirect effects (inhibitory actions) on dorsal raphe nucleus-5HT neurons.

In conclusion, the central components of the stress system, which are located in the hypothalamus and brainstem, can also be considered as parts of the supra-spinal system that provides the excitability command to spinal motoneurons and, possibly, interneurons. Exciting and unanswered questions about the force-producing capacity and motor performance of the skeletal muscles require a better elucidation of the mechanisms underlying both the neuromodulatory control of motoneurons and the generation of dendritic persistent inward currents.

Hormonal Mechanisms Involved in Growth and Remodeling of Skeletal Muscles

It is the nature of almost all hormones to play multiple roles in their physiological functions. However, with respect to the muscular actions, hormones are usually distinguished in anabolic or catabolic mediators of muscle protein metabolism. The following hormones have been classically identified as anabolic: growth hormone (GH), insulin-like growth factors (IGFs), insulin, testosterone, and catecholamines. Moreover, it is becoming increasingly evident that other factors also potentiate skeletal muscle growth. Other hormones (e.g., ghrelin), autocrine/paracrine cytokines (e.g., interleukin-15), and growth factors (e.g., mechano-growth factor and neuregulins) have been implicated in muscle growth in animal and cell culture models. The inhibitory regulators of skeletal muscle growth that were most extensively studied are hormones such as glucocorticoids and angiotensin II, and several cytokines (tumor necrosis factor-α, interleukin-1, and myostatin). Hormones, cytokines, and growth factors that interact with skeletal muscles are part of an integrated system that mediates (and is responsible of) the training-induced adaptations in muscle mass and function: the various components of this integrated system exert their actions through mechanisms taking place in different compartments of the muscle fibers. Therefore, rather than presenting an exhausting catalog of muscular processes regulated by hormones, we aimed to illustrate the complex nature of the integration between different factors involved in muscle growth and remodeling. To do this, we distinguished the different regulators of muscle growth on the basis of the respective site(s)/mechanism(s) of action.

Factors Influencing Protein Synthesis

Glucocorticoids are well-known inhibitors of protein synthesis, primarily in type II (fast-twitch) muscle fibers. The main inhibitory mechanisms include impaired regulation of the activity of nuclear factors involved in peptide initiation (i.e., reduction of the translation efficiency) and inhibition of the antiapoptotic effects of IGFs [11]. Testosterone is considered the primary hormone which interacts with skeletal muscles for cell growth. Its anabolic action can be mediated by different mechanisms: it binds to cytoplasmic receptors to increase protein synthesis and acts as an antiglucocorticoid to suppress protein degradation. In addition, testosterone can also mediate the responses of other anabolic hormones, notably IGFs [12]. Circulating (liver) IGFs and insulin are well-known anabolic factors that have been shown to increase glucose and amino acid uptake, stimulate protein synthesis, and inhibit proteolysis. Their anabolic actions are related to the transcriptional regulation of selected genes. However, circulating IGFs are thought to play a minor role in mediating muscle growth in response to mechanical loading. In fact, most circulating IGFs (>75%) are bound as a ternary complex with IGF binding protein 3 and an acid-labile subunit which apparently does not cross the capillary endothelium. On the contrary, different isoforms of IGF-1 were found to be expressed by muscle fibers in response to stretch and/or loading [13] and/ or GH stimulation [14], and provided the link between mechanical stimuli and the activation of gene expression. One of these isoforms results from an alternative splicing of the IGF-1 gene and has been called mechano-growth factor (MGF) to distinguish it from the liver IGFs which have a systemic mode of action [13]. This autocrine IGF system is also currently under extensive investigation in muscle atrophy research: its impairment has been implicated in muscle protein loss induced by both angiotensin II [15] and proinflammatory cytokines [16]. A muscle-derived factor that complements the anabolic actions of the autocrine IGF system is represented by interleukin-15 (IL-15). IL-5 is a cytokine, highly expressed in skeletal muscle [17], that exerts autocrine and paracrine effects. It stimulated the accumulation of contractile proteins in differentiated muscle cells [17] and stimulated myogenic differentiation independently of IGFs, suggesting that its differentiative activity may be of physiological significance in conditions in which IGF concentrations are low or in which IGFs are sequestered by binding proteins [18]. Finally, catecholamines secreted by the adrenal medulla and norepinephrine released from adrenergic terminals produce anabolic, protein-sparing effects on muscle protein metabolism. These effects seem to be mediated by beta(2)-adrenoceptors and cyclic adenosine monophosphate-dependent pathways, and the underlying mechanisms are inhibition of Ca(2+)-dependent protein degradation and increased rate of protein synthesis in oxidative muscles [19]. In addition, the stimulatory effects of the adrenergic hormones on protein synthesis are potentiated by thyroid hormones [20], which also alter muscle phenotype through the receptor-dependent regulation of responsive genes, namely genes coding for contractile proteins [20].

Factors Regulating Satellite Cells

Satellite cells are mononucleated myoblasts residing in the periphery of muscle fibers [21]; following activation, they proliferate and fuse with muscle fibers and initiate activation of muscle regenerative pathways. MGF and other IGF isoforms act as local tissue repair factors and, following (exercise-induced) damages, are involved in initiating the activation and proliferation of satellite cells [22]. In contrast, a member of the transforming growth factor (TGF)-β family, known as growth and differentiation factor-8 or myostatin [23], inhibits satellite cell proliferation and its downregulation may play a role in fiber hypertrophy [24]. In vivo, differentiation of muscle fibers involves first the MGF-sustained (myostatin-inhibited) expansion of the population of myoblasts and then cell cycle exit and initiation of terminal differentiation, which involves the expression of contractile proteins and the formation of multinucleated syncitia by myocytes fusion. The signals triggering growth arrest and involved in the induction of myoblasts differentiation and fusion still remain to be elucidated. Interestingly, Filigheddu et al. [25] recently found that ghrelin, a GH-releasing peptide with a widespread tissue distribution, induced the differentiation of proliferating myoblasts and promoted their fusion into multinucleated syncitia in vitro.

Factors Affecting Membrane Excitability

The proliferative and metabolic responses of skeletal muscle to contractile activity involve the complex integration of both intra- (muscular) and inter- (neuro-muscular) cellular signal pathways. Neuregulins (NRGs) belong to a complex family of transmembrane proteins [26]. Muscle contractile activity can elicit the expression of multiple NRG isoforms [26]: this can be relevant for the motoneuron–muscle interaction during and after exercise. In fact, NRGs have been implicated in the regulation of synapse formation and maintenance, induction of acetylcholine receptor expression, and maturation of the postsynaptic membrane at the neuro-muscular junction. The depolarization of the postsynaptic membrane is the first and fundamental step of a cascade of events known as excitation–contraction coupling. Factors affecting this coupling can exert relevant influences on muscle performance and adaptations to training. For instance, a suppressive effect of glucocorticoids on sarcolemmal excitability has been reported in few studies [27]: this is possibly due to steroid-induced alterations of sarcolemma permeability. On the contrary, the expression of proteins involved in fluxes of intracellular calcium is upregulated by thyroid hormones, which are known to increase calcium-transport capacity of the sarcoplasmic reticulum [20].

Ultimately, the interactions between hormones and skeletal muscle consequent to training are just starting to be understood from basic research findings. Now the challenge will be the elucidation of the mechanisms that are triggered by "specific" tasks of contraction and types of training.

References

1. Duchateau J, Semmler JG, Enoka RM. Training adaptations in the behavior of human motor units. J Appl Physiol 2006;101:1766–1775.

2. Heckman CJ, Lee RH, Bronstone RM. Hyperexcitable dendrites in motoneurons and their neuromodulatory control during motor behaviour. Trends Neurosci 2003;26:688–695.
3. Brownstone RM. Beginning at the end: repetitive firing properties in the final common pathway. Prog Neurobiol 2006;78:156–172.
4. Chrousos GP. The hypothalamic–pituitary–adrenal axis and immune-mediated inflammation. N Engl J Med 1995;332:1351–1362.
5. Valentino RJ, Foote SL, Page ME. The locus coeruleus as a site for integrating corticotropin-releasing factor and noradrenergic mediation of stress responses. Ann N Y Acad Sci 1993;697: 173–188.
6. Van Bockstaele EJ, Colago EEO, Valentino RJ. Corticotropin-releasing factor-containing axon terminals synapse onto catecholamine dendrites and may presynaptically modulate other afferents in the rostral pole of the nucleus locus coeruleus in the rat brain. J Comp Neurol 1996;364:523–534.
7. Curtis AL, Florin-Lechner SM, Pavcovich LA, et al. Activation of the locus coeruleus noradrenergic system by intracoerulear microinfusion of corticotropin-releasing factor: effects on discharge rate, cortical norepinephrine levels and cortical electroencephalographic activity. J Pharmacol Exp Ther 1997;281:163–172.
8. Sakanaka M, Shibasaki T, Lederis K. Corticotropin releasing factor-like immunoreactivity in the rat brain as revealed by a modified cobalt-glucose oxidase-diaminobenzidine method. J Comp Neurol 1987;260:256–298.
9. Price ML, Curtis AL, Kirby LG, et al. Effects of corticotropin-releasing factor on brain serotonergic activity. Neuropsychopharmacology 1998;18:492–502.
10. Waselus M, Valentino RJ, Van Bockstaele EJ. Ultrastructural evidence for a role of gamma-aminobutyric acid in mediating the effects of corticotropin-releasing factor on the rat dorsal raphe serotonin system. J Comp Neurol 2005;482:155–165.
11. Owczarek J, Jasi ska M, Orszulak-Michalak D. Drug-induced myopathies. An overview of the possible mechanisms. Pharmacol Rep 2005;57:23–34.
12. Wu FC. Endocrine aspects of anabolic steroids. Clin Chem 1997;43:1289–1292.
13. Goldspink G. Changes in muscle mass and phenotype and the expression of autocrine and systemic growth factors by muscle in response to stretch and overload. J Anat 1999;194: 323–334.
14. Kaplan SA, Cohen P. The somatomedin hypothesis 2007: 50 years later. J Clin Endocrinol Metab 2007;92:4529–4535.
15. Brink M, Price SR, Chrast J, et al. Angiotensin II induces skeletal muscle wasting through enhanced protein degradation and down-regulates autocrine insulin-like growth factor I. Endocrinology 2001;142:1489–1496.
16. O'Connor JC, McCusker RH, Strle K, et al. Regulation of IGF-I function by proinflammatory cytokines: at the interface of immunology and endocrinology. Cell Immunol 2008;252:91–110.
17. Quinn LS, Haugk KL, Grabstein KH. Interleukin-15: a novel anabolic cytokine for skeletal muscle. Endocrinology 1995;136:3669–3672.
18. Quinn LS, Haugk KL, Damon SE. Interleukin-15 stimulates C2 skeletal myoblast differentiation. Biochem Biophys Res Commun 1997;239:6–10.
19. Navegantes LC, Migliorini RH, do Carmo Kettelhut I. Adrenergic control of protein metabolism in skeletal muscle. Curr Opin Clin Nutr Metab Care 2002;5:281–286.
20. Simonides WS, van Hardeveld C. Thyroid hormone as a determinant of metabolic and contractile phenotype of skeletal muscle. Thyroid 2008;18:205–216.
21. Chargé SB, Rudnicki MA. Cellular and molecular regulation of muscle regeneration. Physiol Rev 2004;84:209–238.
22. Hill M, Goldspink G. Expression and splicing of the insulin-like growth factor gene in rodent muscle is associated with muscle satellite (stem) cell activation following local tissue damage. J Physiol 2003;549:409–418.
23. McPherron AC, Lawler AM, Lee SJ. Regulation of skeletal muscle mass in mice by a new TGF-beta superfamily member. Nature 1997;387:83–90.

24. Schuelke M, Wagner KR, Stolz LE, et al. Myostatin mutation associated with gross muscle hypertrophy in a child. N Engl J Med 2004;350:2682–2688.
25. Filigheddu N, Gnocchi VF, Coscia M, et al. Ghrelin and des-acyl ghrelin promote differentiation and fusion of C2C12 skeletal muscle cells. Mol Biol Cell 2007;18:986–994.
26. Lebrasseur NK, Coté GM, Miller TA, et al. Regulation of neuregulin/ErbB signaling by contractile activity in skeletal muscle. Am J Physiol Cell Physiol 2003;284:C1149–C1155.
27. van der Hoeven JH. Decline of muscle fiber conduction velocity during short-term high-dose methylprednisolone therapy. Muscle Nerve 1996;19:100–102.

Chapter 8
Sports, Hormones, and Doping in Children and Adolescents

Alan D. Rogol

Introduction

Can one grow more rapidly during childhood and early adolescence and to a taller than genetically programmed adult height or to a more robust body composition given anabolic-androgenic steroids (AAS), human growth hormone (rhGH), insulin-like growth factor (rhIGF-I), insulin, or erythropoietin? Does growth in these dimensions permit an adolescent to reach his/her athletic goals – increased performance – whether faster (citius) in many events, higher (altius) in jumping events, and stronger (fortius)? Why would one consider that possible? The more successful late childhood and early adolescent age athletes are often more physically mature than their age-peers [1]. Early development seemingly permits them to use the strength and power in sport that their average (or even slowly) developing age-peers have not yet attained. The exception to this "rule" might be those athletes in the more esthetic sports in which flexibility and a lower center of gravity are more important than size and strength [1]. These are virtually exclusively in girls.

Most boys' sports require strength and power; however, at higher levels of competition it favors technique as well; for the athlete must produce, control, and efficiently use the energy in a fashion that maximizes sport performance, for example, explosive power in some jumping sports or overall technical skill in the pole vault. Early developing children are taller and stronger than their age-peers. That may confer an advantage at younger ages; however, sport-specific skills are important. It is because of these that some of the "later blooming" adolescents catch up with their earlier developing peers in performance and likely overtake them, for they have had the discipline to attain the requisite skills and are perhaps at lesser risk to "burn-out" and cease participation in that sport.

A.D. Rogol (✉)
Riley Hospital for Children, Indiana University School of Medicine, Indianapolis, IN, USA
and
University of Virginia, Charlottesville, VA, USA
e-mail: adrogol@comcast.net

E. Ghigo et al. (eds.), *Hormone Use and Abuse by Athletes*, Endocrine Updates 29,
DOI 10.1007/978-1-4419-7014-5_8, © Springer Science+Business Media, LLC 2011

Athletics (training and competing) has come to play an increasingly important role in the lives of children and adolescents. With the thousands of dollars spent on coaching, equipment and the possibilities of college scholarships in addition to professional contracts, pediatricians are now being asked to prescribe rhGH and anabolic steroids to attempt to make *normally sized* children and adolescents "better" athletes by making them bigger and stronger. The rationale for taking ergogenic "effectors," such as rhGH and anabolic steroids, is that by becoming bigger and stronger the athlete will perform better. Some boys who are not athletes take anabolic steroids to "look better." However, there are no definitive data for rhGH in young adults and none at all for either rhGH or anabolic steroids in adolescents. Although expensive, rhGH is seemingly little different (if it works to improve athletic performance) from very expensive coaches, equipment, and training camps.

Physiology of Normal Puberty

Physical Changes

Secondary Sexual Characteristics

The method described by Tanner (stages 1–5) is the most widely utilized throughout the world for assessing sexual maturation [2]. The stages are defined by physical characteristics such as the shape and size of the breasts, genitalia, and the development of pubic hair. Breast development is usually the first evidence of puberty in girls, thinning of the scrotum and increased testicular size are usually the first physical signs of puberty among boys. In general, pubertal testicular enlargement has begun when the longitudinal measurement of a testis is greater than 2.5 cm (excluding the epididymis) or the volume is 4 ml or greater [3].

Pubertal Growth Spurt

The pubertal growth spurt can be divided into three stages: the stage of minimal growth velocity just before the spurt (takeoff velocity), the stage of most rapid growth or peak height velocity (PHV), and the stage of diminished velocity and cessation of growth at epiphyseal fusion. Boys reach PHV approximately 2 years later than girls and are taller at takeoff; PHV occurs at stages 3–4 of puberty in most boys and is completed by stage 5 in more than 95% [4, 5]. The mean age at takeoff is 11 years, and the PHV occurs at a mean age of 13.5–14 years in boys. In girls, the mean age at takeoff occurs approximately 2 years earlier. The total height gain in boys between takeoff and cessation of growth is approximately 28 cm. It is approximately 25 cm in girls. Given the slightly less intense growth spurt and the "extra" 2 years of prepubertal growth for boys, one can explain the mean height difference between adult height in men and women of approximately 13 cm.

Bone Age and Body Composition

Skeletal maturation is assessed by comparing radiographs of the hand, the knee, or the elbow with standards of maturation in a normal population [6]. In normal children, bone age, an index of physiological maturation, does not have a precisely defined relationship to the onset of puberty and is as variable as the chronologic age; however, in children with delayed puberty, bone age correlates better with the onset of secondary sexual characteristics than chronologic age.

There are large changes in body composition during puberty in adolescents of both genders; however, they are more dramatic in males and include increases in lean body mass, skeletal mass, bone mineral density, and body water, and decreases in percentage fat mass [7]. In girls, there is an increase in subcutaneous fat mass and a lesser increase in lean body mass. Despite the cessation of linear growth at approximately 15 years in girls and 17 years in boys, neither has attained their adult body composition. That, including peak bone mineral density, does not occur until early in the third decade in females and several years later in males.

Hormonal Changes

Gonadotropins

Before puberty, the pulse amplitude of gonadotropin release is low and occurs infrequently. The onset of pubertal hormonal changes is first evident in dramatic episodes of LH release of short duration that first occur in close proximity to the first episode of deep sleep. With maturity, LH release occurs regularly throughout the day and night [8]. The intermittent release of gonadotropins is reflective of the episodic release of gonadotropin-releasing hormone (GnRH) [9]. The increased sex hormone production by the testes and ovaries results from increased LH stimulation; FSH stimulates the Sertoli cells to initiate spermatogenesis and the ovary to initiate folliculogenesis.

Sex Steroids

Prepubertal boys have plasma testosterone concentrations of less than 0.3 nmol/l (0.1 ng/ml) [8] except during the first 3–5 months of life, when pubertal levels are found. Nighttime elevations of serum testosterone are detectable in the male before the onset of physical signs of puberty and during early puberty after the development of sleep-entrained secretion of LH [8]. In the daytime, testosterone levels begin to increase at approximately 11 years of age, after the testis volume is at least 4 ml, and continue to increase throughout puberty. The steepest increment in testosterone levels occurs between pubertal stages 2 and 3 [10]. A similar rise in estradiol occurs in girls, but several years earlier than testosterone in boys. The nighttime increment in LH stimulates the ovarian follicle to produce estradiol. Early in puberty, these small amounts of estradiol are able to inhibit GnRH release and thus the levels of LH and estradiol are low during the day. This is similar to the changes noted with testosterone in boys; however, the inhibition of LH secretion in boys is also due to estradiol – that is, the rising levels of testosterone are converted in the hypothalamus to estradiol by aromatase. Many actions of testosterone on growth, skeletal maturation, and accretion of bone mass are, to a great extent, the result of its central and peripheral aromatization to estradiol.

Adrenal Androgens

There is a progressive increase in plasma levels of dehydroepiandrosterone (DHEA) and its sulfated form (DHEAS) in both boys and girls that begins by the age of 7 or 8 years and continues throughout early adulthood. The increase in the secretion of adrenal androgens and its precursors is known as "adrenarche" and is independent of the activation of the hypothalamic-pituitary-gonadal axis (gonadarche). The outward sign of increased adrenal androgen production is "pubarche" or the onset of the development of sexual hair – on the pubes or in the axillae.

Growth Hormone, Insulin-Like Growth Factor-I, and Insulin

Serum growth hormone (GH) levels rise during pubertal development in both boys and girls as a result of increased central levels of estradiol (see above). Basal GH secretion is evident before puberty; the amplitude and mass of GH secretion, but not secretory episodes, are increased during pubertal development [7]. This increase in pubertal GH secretion is accompanied by a concomitant rise in plasma insulin-like growth factor-I (IGF-1) levels.

Physiological Role of GH/IGF-I System in Children and Adolescents

The physiological role of hGH is linear growth in children: to promote anabolic (tissue building) metabolism and to alter body composition as part of this anabolic role. Growth hormone actions include the hepatic and local synthesis and release of its main mediator-protein, IGF-I. Its growth-promoting effects include: longitudinal bone growth by actions on the prechondrocytes at the epiphysis. It shares some of these roles with IGF-I, meaning that the direct effect of GH and/or *local* production of IGF-I are both necessary for optimal growth [11]. The direct effects of hGH lead to increased glucose availability, increased free fatty acid levels, and increased amino acid uptake by muscle. Longer-term effects are mediated via IGF-I and include endocrine and importantly paracrine effects in muscle and bone [11]. The outcome of GH *replacement* therapy in a GH-deficient child or adolescent may be an increase in fat-free mass, both body cell mass (muscle), total body water, especially the extra-cellular compartment, a decrease in body fat with a redistribution from central to peripheral [12]. A more detailed analysis of the metabolic effects of GH/IGF-I in exercise is presented in Chap. 2.

Doping with Performance-Enhancing Endocrine Drugs

Definition of Doping

The International Olympic Committee's (IOC) definition of doping is the "*...use of an expedient (substance or method) which is potentially harmful to athletes' health and/or capable of enhancing their performance, or the presence in the athletes' body of a prohibited substance or evidence of the use thereof or evidence of the use of a prohibited method.*" There is no mention of intent or of how the substance entered the body. If the substance is in the athlete's body, then (s)he is responsible. That is the basis of sanctions for testing positive for a prohibited substance. Sir Arthur Porritt, first chairman of the IOC Medical Commission, noted: "*To define doping is, if not impossible, at best extremely difficult, and yet everyone who takes part in competitive sport or who administers it knows exactly what it means. The definition lies not in words but in integrity of character.*"

In fact, there is the desire to be the best, the pressure to win, the attitude that doping is necessary to success, that there are expectations about success at many levels, and later on perhaps financial rewards, such as collegiate scholarships and salary as a professional athlete [13].

Such agents are also known as "performance-enhancing substances" (PES) (Table 8.1). The American Academy of Pediatrics defines these agents as: "*...any substance when taken in nonpharmacological doses specifically for the purposes of improving sport performance. A substance should be considered performance enhancing if it benefits sports performance by increasing strength, power, speed or endurance (ergogenic) or by altering body weight or body composition*" [14]. The agents that will be discussed are those noted in some of the other chapters in this section of this volume: anabolic steroids (and steroid precursors), growth hormone, and erythropoietin (and similar agents). I shall not discuss amino-acids and nonhormonal compounds, for they are among the subjects in the last chapter of this section and there are few (if any) credible data that would distinguish doping from physiology.

Table 8.1 Performance-enhancing substances

Pharmacologic agents (prescription or nonprescription) taken in doses that exceed the
  recommended therapeutic dose or taken when the therapeutic indication(s) are not present
  (e.g., using decongestants for stimulant effect, using bronchodilators when exercise-induced
  bronchospasm is not present, increasing baseline methylphenidate hydrochloride dose
  for athletic competition)
Agents used for weight control, including stimulants, diet pills, diuretics, and laxatives, when
  the user is in a sport that has weight classifications or that rewards leanness
Agents used for weight gain, including over-the-counter products advertised as promoting
  increased muscle mass
Physiologic agents or other strategies used to enhance oxygen-carrying capacity, including
  erythropoietin and red blood cell transfusions (blood doping)
Any substance that is used for reasons other than to treat a documented disease state
  or deficiency
Any substance that is known to mask adverse effects or detectability of another performance-
  enhancing substance
Nutritional supplements taken at supraphysiologic doses or at levels greater than required
  to replace deficits created by a disease state, training, and/or participation in sports

Anabolic Steroids

Adolescents take drugs of abuse for many reasons including as a "rite of passage"
into adulthood. Sport doping may be more specific: improving appearance and/or
augmenting athletic performance. Prevalence data for the nonmedical use of
anabolic steroids have been collected over the past two decades and the data range
from 3 to 8% in boys and 0.5 to 3% in girls in the majority of the surveys [15, 16].
The prevalence of the use of the anabolic steroid precursors, DHEA, androstenedione,
and androstenediol among adolescents is unknown at present [17]. Use in middle
school athletes and among girls has increased at a more rapid rate.

The adverse events for long-term usage are very likely the same as for adults
(Chap. 9), but the doses and duration of use are significantly less in the adolescent than
in the adult. Adverse events unique to, or more severe in, adolescents include acceleration
of pubertal development, early epiphyseal closure and reduced adult height, masculinization
of females, and perhaps *severe* acne. These adverse events depend on the gender of the
athlete, genetic factors, for example, the length of the CAG repeats in the androgen
receptor gene [18] and those related directly to the specific agent: dose, frequency and
duration of exposure, and susceptibility to cause hepatotoxicity (17α-alkylated steroids).
The ergogenic claims are quite difficult to "prove" at least in males, since the effects of
either anabolic steroids or the steroid precursors are those of normal pubertal development.
There is very little difference between the late adolescent and early adult male, for both
continue to accrue lean body mass. The ergogenic claims regarding the prohormone
supplements are not supported by the results of controlled studies (done in adults). There
are convincing data that ingestion of androstenedione leads to increases in circulating
estrogens by peripheral aromatization. The more long-term metabolic effect notes in
adults are discussed in Chap. 9. There should be few significant differences in the
methodology for detection of endogenous or exogenous anabolic steroids (Chap. 13).

Growth Hormone/IGF-I and Insulin to Enhance Athletic Performance

The rationale for taking ergogenic "effectors" such as rhGH, rhIGF-I, and insulin is that by becoming bigger and stronger the athlete will perform better. GH is lipolytic in addition to being anabolic. It should be noted that performance is much more than just strength or endurance, for the athlete must produce, control, and efficiently use the energy in a fashion that maximizes the sport performance.

GH Abuse

GH is listed under class S2 of hormones and related substances in terms of the 2006 World Anti-Doping Agency (WADA) prohibited list. Other peptides in this category include erythropoietin (EPO) and corticotrophin (ACTH) in addition to IGF-I and insulin, itself [19]. GH is likely being abused at an increasingly prevalent rate, but before describing some of the data, it should be noted that much of what is purported to be hGH, especially as found on the internet, is not. Of course, any drug taken orally cannot be hGH. Liu et al. [20] have systematically reviewed the effects of rhGH on athletic performance mainly in young adults. The main points of that review were:

- Very few studies evaluated strength and exercise capacity.
- Small effects would not have been found.
- Short duration of the studies, many for only one dose.
- Doses of rhGH and other "supplements" are very likely different in the "real world" of the athlete.

These investigators concluded: *"Claims regarding the performance-enhancing properties of growth hormone are premature and are not supported by our review of the literature. The limited published data evaluating the effects of growth hormone on athletic performance suggest that although growth hormone increases lean body mass in the short term, it does not appear to improve strength and may worsen exercise capacity. In addition, growth hormone in the healthy young is frequently associated with adverse events"* [20].

Abuse of IGF-I is more recent than that of rhGH. It is likely to be of much lower prevalence and its effects (and adverse events) are less well known than those for rhGH. There are no credible data in adolescent athletes, but the most serious adverse event, hypoglycemia, is likely much less than in children with GH insensitivity, since the former will have a greater circulating concentration of IGFBP-3, the major binding protein for IGF-I and acid-labile subunit, the third member of the circulating ternary complex for IGF-I. This complex diminishes the concentration of "free" (unbound IGF-I) and its hypoglycemia potential. Other adverse events include some of those for rhGH – edema, headache, arthralgia, and jaw pain [21]. Although there is no specific test to detect doping with IGF-I, it would appear that the approach using pharmacodynamic markers as done for rhGH (Chap. 15) will be appropriate with the caveat that the normal values depend on gender and stage of adolescent development. Since adolescents, including athletes, may be in different stages of pubertal development at *any* chronological age, the normal values will have a very broad range, making it difficult to interpret a single value for an individual and thus even more difficult to detect doping in the younger athletes.

Insulin is a potent anabolic agent. It leads to weight gain through at least two actions: it is lipogenic and it inhibits protein breakdown. It is likely used much more than stated in the literature, for it is inexpensive, readily available, and virtually undetectable for doping purposes. Its most common side effect is hypoglycemia for which athletes take additional carbohydrate at the time that they inject the short-acting insulin. However, it should be noted that virtually anyone receiving insulin will have some immunological reaction and those using the newer insulin analogs will have traces of the noninsulin portions of the molecules that make them longer acting [22].

Erythropoietin (EPO)

EPO is a circulating glycosylated protein hormone that is the principal regulator of erythropoiesis. It is produced primarily by the kidney in relationship to the concentration of O_2 in the blood. Following administration, there is a direct relationship between hemoglobin levels and increased performance following administration of rHuEPO in rats and humans [23]. Proper clinical use of EPO, erythropoiesis-stimulating agents, and other methods to enhance oxygen transport should diminish the need for blood transfusion, and enhance resting energy levels, tolerance to physical exercise, and the sense of well being. All are commonly noted in patients with severe anemia secondary to chronic kidney disease, cancer and its chemotherapy, or other diseases.

Methods used in doping include hypoxia and hypoxia-mimetics. One such method is to train at altitude; however, one cannot necessarily train as hard as at lower altitude because of hypoxic-mediated fatigue. Variations on this theme include living at altitude and training at sea level or sleeping in a tent or chamber with diminished oxygen tension (at lower altitude) and training at the same elevation. These methods are not considered doping. Blood and blood substitutes (for example, perfluorocarbons) are considered doping and both may have significant toxicities. Homologous blood transfusions require proper storage and autologous ones can lead to transfusion reactions. The blood substitutes have unfavorable O_2 dissociation kinetics as well as toxicities of their own, including vasoconstriction.

rHuEPO and its follow-on biological relatives can provide an effective mechanism to stimulate erythropoiesis as noted above; however, the baseline hematocrit increases and may rise even more to dangerous levels, likely due to dehydration, in athletes during and after training and competition. The rheology of blood changes exponentially as the hematocrit rises above 55% and accelerates even more rapidly as it rise above 60%. Deaths in competitive cyclists have been directly linked to this phenomenon. Gene doping with EPO (see below) may be problematic either because of the death of the cells to which the gene has been transferred and perhaps uncontrolled release of EPO with its attendant marked increase in hemoglobin levels.

There are no studies of rHuEPO, or its related proteins in childhood or adolescent athletes, but theoretically there should be no difference in the responses from older adolescents or young adults. The major issues are those that relate to increased hematocrit-sluggish blood flow in the small vessels of critical organs and pulmonary emboli. Theoretically, similar arguments may be made for the transfusion of homologous or autologous blood and the blood substitutes, but there are no available data.

Other erythropoiesis-stimulating agents include Hematide, a novel peptide-based erythropoietin-mimetic [24], CERA (Continuous Erythropoietin Receptor Activator), a large peptide related to EPO [25], and hypoxia-inducible factor (HIF) stabilizers which are orally active compounds that inhibit the prolyl hydroxylase that degrades HIF, permitting upregulation of EPO gene expression [26]. All are in stages of development for various anemias and there are no data in athletes, although all should increase erythropoiesis and thus are at risk for use by athletes.

Gene Doping

The era of gene doping, for example, adding hGH or hIGF-I genes to specific muscles, has arrived. Experiments have been done in animals [27]. No detection methods presently available could detect this type of doping. To protect athletes from this presently theoretical concern, the WADA has declared that "the non-therapeutic use of cells, genes, genetic elements, or the modulation of gene expression, having the capacity to enhance athletic performance, is prohibited" [28]. Candidate molecules for this approach might include: GH and IGF-I and some of its isoforms (splice variants), including mechano growth factor [29]. Administration of mechano growth factor to older mice permitted the muscles to maintain hypertrophy and to regenerate in a physiologic manner, as if the muscles were from younger animals.

Myostatin is a negative regulator or muscle mass and has been noted to be inactive in "over-muscled" animals and in a single child [30]. Doping to gain advantage would be aimed at inactivating myostatin biological activity.

Other genes whose alteration might enhance athletic performance include: EPO, vascular endothelial growth factor, and a number of the peroxisome-proliferator-activated receptor (PPAR's). The PPAR-δ isoform has the potential to alter the proportion of oxidative slow twitch fibers in muscle [31, 32].

None of these possibilities (and likely many more) is ready for use in the human; however, there will be major technical hurdles with the products and procedures (viral vectors, especially their uncontrolled growth; liposomes) and specific ones for each of the proteins transferred, for example, the induction of tumors with hGH or IGF-I or one of its isoforms; the increase in hematocrit with EPO; and the altered blood rheology. Detection by present methods is particularly unlikely and that may push athletes to this relatively untested procedure. The short half-lives of the secreted proteins would make the detection of these substances difficult. It may be that pharmacodynamic markers, as presently used for rhGH, immune responses to the viral vectors, or physical methods to detect parts of the liposomes would be the direction toward which the doping detection process would turn.

References

1. Malina RM, Bouchard C, Bar-Or O. The young athlete. In: Malina RM, Bouchard C, Bar-Or O, editors. Growth, Maturation and Physical Activity, 2nd edition. Human Kinetics Press, Champaign, IL, 2004, pp 623–49.
2. Tanner JM. Growth at Adolescence. Springfield, Charles C. Thomas, 1962.
3. Zachmann M, Prader A, Kind HP, et al. Testicular volume during adolescence: cross-sectional and longitudinal studies. Helv Paediatr Acta. 1974; 29:61–72.
4. Tanner JM, Whitehouse RH, Marubini E, Resele LF. The adolescent growth spurt of boys and girls of the Harpenden growth study. Ann Hum Biol. 1976; 3:109–26.
5. Largo RH. Analysis of the adolescent growth spurt using smoothing spline function. Ann Hum Biol. 1978; 5:421–34.
6. Greulich WS, Pyle SI. Radiograph Atlas of Skeletal Development of the Hand and Wrist. Stanford: Stanford University Press, 1959.
7. Veldhuis JD, Roemmich JN, Richmind EJ, et al. Endocrine control of body composition in infancy, childhood, and puberty. Endocr Rev. 2005; 26:114–46.
8. Albertsson-Wikland K, Rosberg S, Lannering B, et al. Twenty-four-hour profiles of luetinizing hormone, follicle-stimulating hormone, testosterone, and estradiol levels: a semi-longitudinal study throughout puberty in healthy boys. J Clin Endocrinol Metab. 1997; 82:541–9.
9. Knobil E. The neuroendocrine control of the menstrual cycle. Recent Prog Horm Res. 1980; 36:53–88.
10. Knorr D. Plasma testosterone in male puberty. 1. Physiology of plasma testosterone. Acta Endocrinol (Copenh). 1974; 75:181–94.
11. Melmed S, Klineberg D. Anterior pituitary. In: Kronenberg HM, Melmed S, Polonsky KS, Larsen PR, editors. Williams Textbook of Endocrinology, 11th edition. Sanders (Elsevier), New York, 2008, pp 155–261.
12. Roemmich, JN, Huerta MG, Sundaresan SM, Rogol AD. Alterations in body composition and fat distribution in growth hormone deficient prepubertal children during growth hormone therapy. Metabolism. 2001; 50:537–47.
13. Holland-Hall C. Performance-enhancing substances: is your adolescent patient using? Pediatr Clin N Am. 2007; 54:651–62.
14. American Academy of Pediatrics Committee on Sports Medicine and Fitness. Use of performance-enhancing substances. Pediatrics. 2005; 115:1103–6.
15. Carpenter PC. Performance-enhancing drugs in sport. Endocrinol Metab Clin N Am. 2007; 36:481–95.
16. Castillo EM, Comstock RD. Prevalence of use of performance-enhancing substances among United States adolescents. Pediatr Clin N Am. 2007; 54:66375.
17. Smurawa TM, Congeni JA. Testosterone precursors: use and abuse in pediatric athletes. Pediatr Clin N Am. 2007; 54:787–96.
18. Zitzmann M, Nieschlag E. The CAG repeat polymorphism within the androgen receptor gene and maleness. Int J Androl. 2003; 26:76–83.
19. World Anti-Doping Agency. http://www.wada-ama.org/, accessed Jan 03, 2009.
20. Liu H, Bravata DM, Okin I, et al. Systematic review: the effects of growth hormone on athletic performance. Ann Int Med. 2008; 144:747–58.
21. Richmond EJ, Rogol AD. Recombinant human insulin-like growth factor-I therapy for children with growth disorders. Adv Ther. 2008; 25:1276–87.

22. Thomas A, Thevis M, Delahaut P, et al. Mass spectrometric identification of degradation products of insulin and its long-acting analogues in human urine for doping control purposes. Anal Chem. 2007; 79:2518–24.
23. Elliott S. Erythropoiesis-stimulating agents and other methods to enhance oxygen transport. Brit J Pharmacol. 2008; 154:529–41.
24. Macdougall IC. Hematide, a novel peptide-based erythopoiesis-stimulating agent for the treatment of anemia. Curr Opin Investig Drugs. 2008; 9:1034–47.
25. Topf JM. CERA: third generation erythropoiesis-stimulating agent. Expert Opin Pharmacother. 2008; 9:839–49.
26. Bunn HF. New agents that stimulate erythropoiesis. Blood. 2007; 109:868–73.
27. Barton-Davis ER, Shoturma DI, Musaro A, et al. Viral mediated expression of insulin-like growth factor I blocks the aging-related loss of skeletal muscle function. Proc Natl Acad Sci USA. 1998; 95:15603–7.
28. Wells DJ. Gene doping: the hype and the reality. Brit J Pharmacol. 2008; 154:623–31.
29. Goldspink G, Yang SY, Hameed M, et al. The role of MGF and other IGF-I splice variants in muscle maintenance and hypertrophy. In: Kraemer WJ and Rogol AD, editors. The Endocrine System in Sports and Exercise. Vol XI, The Encyclopaedia of Sports Medicine, an IOC Medical Commission Publication. Blackwell Publishing, Malden, MA, 2005, pp 180–93.
30. Joulia-Ekaza D, Cabello G. The myostatin gene: physiology and pharmacological relevance. Curr Opin Pharmacol. 2007; 7:310–5.
31. Kraemer DK, Ahlsen M, Norrbom J, et al. Human skeletal muscle fibre type variations correlate with PPAR alpha, PPAR delta and PGC-1 alpha mRNA. Acta Physiol (Oxf). 2007; 188:207–16.
32. Wang YX, Zhang CL, Yu RT, et al. Regulation of muscle fiber type and running endurance by PPARdelta. PLoS Biol. 2004; 2:e294.

Chapter 9
Androgen Abuse

Karen Choong, Ravi Jasuja, Shehzad Basaria, Thomas W. Storer, and Shalender Bhasin

Introduction

The decade of the 1930s was marked by two notable milestones in Endocrinology: the discovery of testosterone as the predominant androgen in humans and its chemical synthesis; these discoveries ushered in the era of the rational hormone replacement therapy of androgen-deficient men. However, two powerful myths have pervaded the academic community for more than seven decades. First, in spite of compelling empiric evidence from the experience of athletes and recreational body builders worldwide, the academic community continued to assert that androgens do not increase muscle mass or strength [1]. Fortunately, this view point has undergone a sea change during the last 10 years as a large number of controlled randomized trials and their meta-analyses, reviewed below, have established unequivocally that testosterone administration is associated with gains in skeletal muscle mass, muscle size, and maximal voluntary strength [2, 3]. The second misperception, widely shared among athletes, sports medicine physicians, and academic endocrinologists is that androgen abuse by athletes and recreational body builders is associated with relatively low frequency of adverse health consequences.

In the world of competition and sports, the use of ergogenic substances by athletes continues to be a growing problem and androgens are among the most frequently abused drugs. Senator Mitchell's report was a tacit acknowledgement of what had been widely known in the sports communities – that the use of performance enhancing drugs by athletes is far more prevalent than anyone is willing to admit [4–6]. A number of professional societies have published position statements condemning the pervasive abuse of androgens in sports [7, 8]; however, these position statements have done little to reduce the high prevalence rates of androgen abuse.

S. Bhasin (✉)
Boston Claude D. Pepper Older Americans Independence Center for Function Promoting Therapies, Section of Endocrinology, Diabetes, and Nutrition, Boston University, School of Medicine, Boston, MA 02118, USA
e-mail: bhasin@bu.edu; Shalender.Bhasin@bmc.org

E. Ghigo et al. (eds.), *Hormone Use and Abuse by Athletes*, Endocrine Updates 29, DOI 10.1007/978-1-4419-7014-5_9, © Springer Science+Business Media, LLC 2011

The history of the evolution of androgen abuse in professional sports has been chronicled in several reviews and will only be mentioned briefly [7, 9–17]. German soldiers were allegedly given anabolic steroids to enhance performance and endurance during combat in World War II. The earliest documented use of anabolic steroids in the history of sports was allegedly by German athletes in the 1936 Berlin Olympics, and later by Russian weightlifters in the Olympics Games of 1952 and 1956 [17]. Dr. John Ziegler, a physician with the US Weight Lifting Team learned about the use of androgens by Russian weight lifters and later administered dianabol to himself and other weight lifters. The androgen abuse by athletes has continued to increase since then. The International Olympic Committee (IOC) introduced antidoping regulations for the first time in 1967, and performed the first antidoping testing in the 1972 Munich Olympics. It was not until 1976 that androgens were placed on the IOC doping list.

Prevalence of Androgen Use

Androgen abuse is frequent in both competitive and recreational sports but the exact prevalence of androgen abuse is difficult to determine as surveys of androgen abuse depend on self-report [17]. An estimated one million Americans had used androgens sometime in their lives, accounting for approximately 1% of the US population. Other countries, such as Canada and Australia, have also witnessed a similar trend. Men tend to have a higher tendency to use androgens as compared to women. The risk factors for androgen abuse include being male, participation in intercollegiate athletics, cigarette smoking, alcohol abuse, and other illicit drug use.

The Monitoring the Future National Survey Results on Drug Use in high school students estimated the prevalence of androgen abuse in 2008 to be 1.5% among 12th graders [18]. The androgen use was more prevalent in boys (1.2, 1.4, and 2.5% among male 8th, 10th, and 12th graders, respectively) than in girls (0.5, 0.5, and 0.4% among female 8th, 10th, and 12th graders, respectively) [18]. Among adults aged 19–30 years, the prevalence rates of androgen use were 1.2% in men and 0.2% in women (*Monitoring the Future Study in college students and adults* [19, 20]).

The use of androgens among high school students has been declining since 2001 from 2.4% of 12th graders in 2001 to 1.5% in 2008; this decrease in androgen use among high school students has been attributed to the negative portrayal of androgen use among professional athletes and of the unfavorable consequences it imposes on their professional careers.

Patterns of Androgen Use

Nandrolone, testosterone, stanozolol, methandienone, and methenolol are the most frequently abused androgens and account for a major fraction of androgen abuse [21–23]. Athletes use intramuscular injections of androgens far more frequently than oral formulations [7, 21]. Also, combinations of androgens are used more frequently than single agents [7, 21, 23]. Multiple androgens may be combined in a practice known as stacking, in which two or more androgens are added in progressively increasing doses over a period of several weeks.

The doses of testosterone or other androgens used by athletes are substantially larger than those prescribed for the treatment of androgen deficiency. In one survey [21], 50% of androgenic steroid users reported using at least 500 mg of testosterone weekly or an equivalent dose of another androgenic steroid; in other surveys [23], 10–25% androgen users reported administration of 1,000 mg testosterone enanthate weekly or an equivalent dose of other androgens.

Athletes also often use a practice called "cycling," in which weeks of androgen use are followed by periods of drug holiday; this routine is based on the unproven premise that cycling prevents desensitization to massive doses of androgen [7]. Building a pyramid refers to the progressive increase in the doses of androgens during a cycle [7]. Towards the end of a cycle, athletes may reduce the doses of androgens or switch to other drugs, such as hCG or aromatase inhibitors or estrogen antagonists, that they believe will reduce the likelihood of testicular suppression [7]. The median cycle length is 11 weeks and a typical androgen stack includes three androgens [21, 24, 25].

Athletes and recreational body builders, who abuse androgens, also abuse other drugs to enhance muscle building, muscle shaping, or athletic performance, and to reduce one or more side effects of androgens [21, 24, 25]. Other drugs that are often abused concomitantly include other anabolic agents such as recombinant human growth hormone, IGF-1, insulin and erythropoietin, stimulants, such as amphetamine, clenbuterol, ephedrine, and thyroxine, and drugs that are perceived to reduce adverse effects such as hCG, aromatase inhibitors, or estrogen antagonists [7, 21, 24, 25].

Effectiveness of Androgens in Increasing Muscle Mass, Muscle Strength, and Athletic Performance

The academicians have long been skeptical of the claims of the anabolic effects of androgens [1]; this skepticism was based on the lack of conclusive experimental evidence and contradictory results from studies performed prior to 1990s. Most studies performed in the past were neither randomized nor blinded. These studies did not standardize energy or protein intake. In some studies, the participants were allowed to ingest protein supplements. The physical activity and training intensity were not controlled; thus, these studies were unable to separate out the effects of resistance exercise training from those of androgen use. Moreover, the doses of androgens used in clinical trials were generally small and insufficient to produce detectable anabolic effects. In contrast athletes who abuse anabolic steroids often administer supraphysiologic doses of multiple androgens.

In the 1990s, a number of studies, some in healthy volunteers and many in androgen-deficient men, turned the tide and established conclusively that androgens increase muscle mass. A number of open-label trials demonstrated that testosterone replacement of healthy hypogonadal young men increases fat-free mass and muscle strength [26–30]. Likewise, suppression of serum testosterone with a GnRH analog in healthy young men resulted in decreases in fat-free mass, fractional muscle protein synthesis, and muscle strength [31]. However, the most compelling evidence emerged from a randomized, placebo-controlled trial [32] that demonstrated that supraphysiologic doses of testosterone enanthate (600 mg intramuscularly) increased skeletal muscle mass (Fig. 9.1). In this study, healthy eugonadal young men (age 19–34 years) were administered either testosterone enanthate (600 mg intramuscularly weekly, six to eight times the replacement dose) or placebo injections with and without a standardized program of progressive, resistance exercise training for a period of 10 weeks. The protein and energy intake were standardized at 1.5 g/kg/day and 40 Kcal/kg/day, respectively [32]. The exercise stimulus was based on the initial 1-RM strength and was clamped at the outset [32]. To minimize the learning effect, only men with prior strength training experience were included. Testosterone administration and resistance exercise were each associated with greater increments in fat-free mass, muscle size, and maximal voluntary strength than placebo. Moreover, the effects of testosterone administration and resistance exercise training combined were greater than those of either intervention alone [32]. Several other trials using supraphysiologic doses of testosterone have confirmed these findings [33].

In subsequent studies, we demonstrated that the gains in skeletal muscle mass and maximal voluntary muscle strength during androgen administration are correlated with androgen dose [34]. When healthy young men (age 18–34 years), whose endogenous testosterone production had been suppressed by administration of a long-acting GnRH agonist, were given graded doses of testosterone enanthate (25, 50, 125, 300, and 600 mg), there was a dose-dependent increase in fat-free mass, muscle size, and maximal voluntary strength [34]. In multivariate analyses, testosterone dose and increments in testosterone concentrations above baseline were the most important predictors of gains in skeletal muscle mass and strength [35].

A number of other randomized clinical trials have shown that testosterone therapy also increases fat-free mass and muscle strength in HIV-infected men with weight loss [36–38] and men with chronic obstructive lung disease [39]. Similar anabolic effects on fat-free mass have been reported in older men with low or low normal testosterone levels [40–42].

Thus, a consensus has emerged that testosterone administration dose-dependently increases skeletal muscle mass, maximal voluntary strength, and leg power. The gains in maximal voluntary strength are proportional to the increments in muscle mass so that the specific force does not change [43]; thus, androgens do not improve the contractile properties of the skeletal muscle. Therefore, it is easy to understand why androgen abuse is most prevalent among weight lifters or among athletes whose performance is dependent upon muscle strength. However, androgens have not been shown to improve measures of whole body endurance, such as VO2max or lactate threshold. Therefore, androgen abuse by athletes who participate in endurance sports such as cycling and sprinting is difficult to understand.

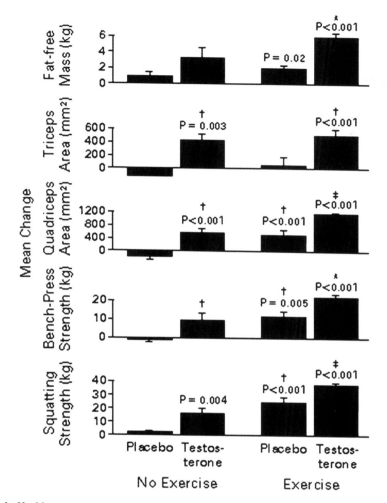

Fig. 9.1 Healthy young men were randomized to receive placebo alone, testosterone enanthate 600 mg intramuscularly weekly, placebo plus progressive resistance exercise training, or testosterone enanthate 600 mg plus progressive resistance exercise training. Treatment duration was 10 weeks. The data are mean ± SEM change from baseline in each of the outcomes shown in the figure above. *P* values relative to zero change are shown. *Dagger: P* value compared to placebo, no exercise group. *Double dagger: P* value relative to testosterone, no exercise group. Reproduced with permission from N Engl J Med

Also, widespread use of androgens by baseball players is also not easily explained. Testosterone increases red blood cell mass and this may increase the oxygen carrying capacity of blood [44]. Testosterone improves neuromuscular transmission and may reduce reaction time [45–47]. It is also possible that testosterone may improve hand eye coordination. Improved hand eye coordination and reaction time could be beneficial to baseball players. It also has been speculated that androgens may allow athletes to train harder by promoting recovery of skeletal muscle between training sessions. These hypotheses have not been tested rigorously.

Mechanisms of Androgen Action

Testosterone induces hypertrophy of type I and type II skeletal muscle fibers in a dose-dependent manner [48–50]. The absolute number or the relative proportion of type I and type II muscle fibers is not affected by testosterone administration [48]. Satellite cells are muscle progenitor cells that are located between the plasma membrane and the basal lamina of muscle fibers and play a key role in muscle fiber hypertrophy. Testosterone administration increases the number of myonuclei and satellite cells (Fig. 9.2) [51]. However, the myonuclear domain does not change significantly.

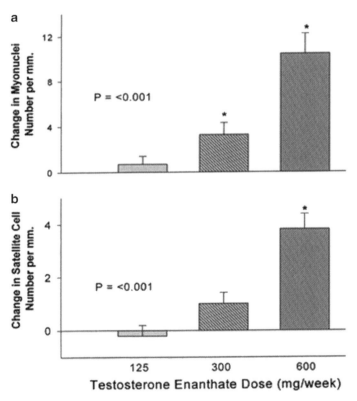

Fig. 9.2 Change from baseline in myonuclear and satellite cell number in vastus lateralis of healthy young men treated with a long-acting GnRH agonist and graded doses of testosterone enanthate for 20 weeks. Data are mean ± SEM. *Asterisk*: $P < 0.05$ relative to zero change. Adapted with permission from [51]

The anabolic effects of androgens are primarily mediated through the androgen receptor (AR)-signaling. Androgen receptors are expressed in the satellite cells and other stem-like cells in the interstitium of the skeletal muscle fibers [52]. Blocking androgen action by androgen receptor antagonists, such as flutamide, reduces fat-free mass. Similarly, mice with muscle specific knock out of androgen receptor have decreased muscle mass [53, 54].

The molecular mechanisms of anabolic effects of androgen on the skeletal muscle remain poorly understood. A growing body of evidence supports the hypothesis that testosterone and dihydrotestosterone promote myogenic differentiation of mesenchymal, multipotent stem cells and inhibit their differentiation into the adipogenic lineage [55–57]. In cultures of mesenchymal multipotent C3H10T1/2 cells, androgens upregulate the expression of myogenic differentiation, MyoD, and myosin heavy chain (MHC) mRNA [57] and down regulate expression of adipogenic differentiation markers, PPAR-gamma, and C/EBP-alpha [55, 56]. Moreover, these actions of testosterone on myogenic differentiation were blocked by bicalutamide (an AR-antagonist) administration [55–57], suggesting an essential role of AR in mediating these effects.

Androgen binding to AR induces specific conformational changes in the receptor [58] and promotes its association with β-catenin and translocation of the AR–β-catenin complex into the nucleus where it associates with TCF-4 [57]. β-catenin plays an essential role in mediating the effects of testosterone on myogenesis because blocking beta-catenin by using siRNAs blocks testosterone's effects on myogenic differentiation [57]. Testosterone activates a number of Wnt target genes, such as follistatin, a potent inhibitor of the action of myostatin and other TGFbeta family members [57]. Smad7 expression, an inhibitory transducer of TGF-B signaling (of which myostatin is a member) is also upregulated by testosterone [57].

Testosterone supplementation has been shown to increase nitrogen retention in castrated males of many mammalian species [59, 60]. Recently, testosterone has been reported to increase fractional muscle protein synthesis and to increase the reutilization of amino acids by the skeletal muscle [27, 61–63]. The effects of testosterone on muscle protein degradation are not well understood. Studies conducted in 1970s suggested that androgens might exert an anti-glucocorticoid effect.

Adverse Effects of Androgen Abuse (Table 9.1)

Given the high prevalence of androgen abuse, the paucity of data on the adverse effects of androgen abuse is indeed remarkable. Much of the literature comprises of either case reports or small retrospective studies based largely on self-reported data [7, 64–67]. Systematic investigations of the adverse effects of androgens in athletes and recreational body builders have been difficult for many reasons. Because of the illicit nature of androgen abuse and the potential for adverse professional consequences in the event of detection, the adverse effects are under reported.

Table 9.1 Potential adverse effects associated with androgen use

Potential adverse effects of high doses of androgens
  Behavioral and psychiatric side effects:
    Increased risk of suicidal and homicidal death
    Depression
    Hypomania and mania
    Increased risk of the use of stimulants and psychoactive drugs,
      and accessories such as hCG, clomiphene, and aromatase inhibitors
  Cardiovascular complications:
    Lowering of HDL cholesterol
    Increased LDL cholesterol
    Sudden cardiac death
    Myocardial hypertrophy and dysfunction
  Prolonged suppression of hypothalamic–pituitary–testicular axis
  Hepatic dysfunction, neoplasms, and peliosis hepatic
  Gynecomastia
  Acne and increased hair growth
  Sexual dysfunction
  Tendon, ligament, and joint injuries
Potential adverse effects of intramuscular injections
  Local infection and abscess
  Systemic infection, including HIV and HCV
Unique adverse effects associated with androgen use in women
  Hirsutism
  Clitoral enlargement
  Change of body habitus, including widening of upper body torso
  Breast atrophy
  Menstrual irregularity
Unique adverse effects associated with androgen use in children
  Premature epiphyseal fusion and growth retardation
  Premature virilization in boys and masculinization in girls
  Increased risk of unhealthy behaviors:
    Use of alcohol, tobacco, and other drugs
    Less frequent seatbelt use
    More sexual activity
    Antisocial behavior
    Declining academic performance
    More fasting, vomiting, diet pill, and laxative use by young girls

Adapted from [64]

These analyses of adverse events are further complicated by the substantial variability in the dose, frequency, duration, and the type of drugs used. The concomitant use of other drugs – stimulants and depressants, and drugs perceived to reduce the risk of adverse effects – renders the attribution of adverse effects to a specific drug difficult. Because most androgen users are athletes or recreational body builders, it is difficult to extricate the effects of androgen use from those of the athletic training. For instance, it is unclear whether the myocardial hypertrophy and tendon injuries reported in some power athletes are due to the effects of androgens or strength training or both.

Widespread perception that these drugs are "not too dangerous" has contributed to a sense of complacency among sports organizations, recreational body builders, and athletes [6]. The low frequency of adverse effects observed in controlled clinical trials of testosterone and other androgens has further fueled this false perception [3]. The data from randomized clinical trials, most of which have used replacement doses of testosterone, should not be extrapolated to the setting of androgen abuse by athletes. The clinical trials of androgens have used substantially lower doses of androgens than those used by athletes and recreational body builders. For instance, the typical dose of testosterone used in testosterone replacement trials is 200 mg every 2 weeks or 5–10 mg of testosterone delivered by testosterone gel or patch; the highest dose of testosterone enanthate used in clinical trials has been 600 mg weekly. In contrast, androgen users in one survey reported using as much as 1,000 mg of testosterone enanthate or more weekly [24]. Furthermore, the vast majority of individuals who abuse androgen also use other drugs; e.g., in one survey 25% of androgen users used growth hormone or insulin [24]. Individuals with certain behavioral and psychiatric disorders may be overrepresented among androgen abusers [68]; these underlying behavioral and psychiatric disorders may render these individuals more susceptible to certain behavioral and psychiatric side effects of androgens. Also, individuals who abuse androgens may engage in high-risk behaviors that may increase the risks of HIV infection, injury, or violence. Therefore, the adverse effects of androgen abuse in individuals predisposed to high-risk behaviors should be viewed differently from those of replacement doses of testosterone in men with low or low normal testosterone levels. To the extent randomized controlled trials of high doses of androgens in athletes or recreational body builders will never be conducted, the information about the adverse effects of androgens of abuse must necessarily be collected from current users, which is an enormously challenging task. Therefore, prospective registries of androgen users to systematically record the health effects of androgens are urgently needed.

The adverse effects associated with androgen abuse can be categorized as follows [7, 21, 24, 33, 66]: the adverse effects attributable to androgens themselves; the adverse effects due to concomitant use of accessory drugs; adverse consequences of androgen withdrawal; and personality and behavioral disorders that render individuals more susceptible to androgen abuse or to adverse effects of androgens. The most frequent side effects reported by individuals using androgens for nonmedical reasons include acne, increased body hair and sex drive, and aggression [21, 24]. Other adverse events that have been reported in association with androgen abuse include mood and psychiatric disorders [23], increased risk of suicidal or homicidal death [69], deleterious changes in the cardiovascular risk factors, including a marked decrease in plasma HDL cholesterol level [70–72] and changes in clotting factors [73], suppression of the hypothalamic–pituitary–testicular axis and spermatogenesis resulting in infertility, and increase in liver enzymes [74–76].

Cutaneous Side Effects of Androgens

Androgen use is associated with acne, male pattern baldness, as well as increased body hair [24, 77]. Some androgen users report increased perspiration.

Androgen Abuse and Mortality

Anecdotal reports and retrospective analyses have suggested higher death rates at remarkably young age among androgen users. For instance, one study compared mortality and underlying causes of mortality among 62 power lifters who had achieved the top five positions in weightlifting competitions in the 82.5–125.0 kg weight categories during the 1977–1982 period to a reference group that included age-matched, individuals from the general population. Thirteen percent of power lifters and 3% of the age-matched control group died during this period. The causes of death among power lifters included suicides, myocardial infarction, hepatic coma, and non-Hodgkin's lymphoma. The risk of death among the power lifters was 4.6 times higher than in the control population. In another study, the median age of death among androgen users who died and were autopsied was 24.5 years [78]; this remarkably young age of death among androgen users is even lower than that for heroin or amphetamine users [78]. A retrospective review of patient records in Sweden [79] also reported substantially higher standardized mortality ratios for androgen users than for patients who were not using androgens.

Among 34 androgen users whose deaths were investigated medicolegally, Thiblin et al. [80] found that 32% had committed suicide, 26% were victims of homicide, and 35% of deaths were deemed accidental [80]. Use of multiple drugs, cardiac causes, and impulsive and uncontrolled violent behaviors were among the contributory causes of accidental deaths [80].

Depressive or hypomania-like symptoms, acts of violence, and/or interpersonal difficulties at work or in personal life have been noted in the period immediately preceding suicide among androgen users [81]. Concomitant abuse of other psycho-active drugs is common among androgen users who die prematurely [78].

Cardiovascular Effects of Androgens

Androgens affect lipoprotein profile, myocardial mass and function, cardiac remodeling, and the risk of thrombosis [82–88]. Several potential mechanisms have been proposed to explain the adverse cardiovascular effects of androgens [82]. High doses of androgens may induce proatherogenic dyslipidemia, increase the risk of thrombosis through their effects on clotting factors and platelets, induce vasospasm through their effects on vascular nitric oxide, or induce myocardial injury because of their direct effects on myocardial cells [82].

The effects on plasma lipids and lipoproteins depend upon the dose of androgen, the route of administration (oral or parenteral), and whether the androgen is aromatizable or not [2, 3, 89–95]. Replacement doses of testosterone, when administered parenterally, are associated with a small decrease in plasma HDL cholesterol levels and little or no effect on total cholesterol, LDL cholesterol, and triglyceride levels [3, 29, 94, 95], but supraphysiologic doses of testosterone even when administered parenterally markedly decrease HDL cholesterol [32, 96]. In contrast, orally administered, 17-alpha-alylated, nonaromatizable androgens produce greater reductions in plasma HDL cholesterol levels and greater increments in LDL cholesterol than parenterally administered testosterone [97].

Most studies have reported either no change or small and transient increases in blood pressure during androgen administration, but some studies have reported large increases in blood pressure in strength athletes.

Many studies of cardiac function, some using echocardiography, have been published. Most of the studies included power lifters or body builders and found no significant changes in left ventricular mass or function. Others have found increases in left ventricular mass, left ventricular posterior wall thickness, interventricular septal thickness, and left ventricular end diastolic volume among androgen users [82, 84–86, 98–100]. Power athletes who use androgens have been reported to have significant impairment of both systolic and diastolic function [98, 101]. Urhausen et al. [102] measured left ventricular mass and wall thickness in power lifters and body builders who were using androgens or had used androgens in the past, and weight lifters who had never used androgens. Current androgen users had higher left ventricular muscle mass than nonusers or previous users [102]. The E/A ratio, a measure of left ventricular diastolic function, is reduced in power lifters using androgens suggesting diastolic dysfunction [103]. Large doses of androgens may increase the risk of heart failure and fibrosis [82, 84, 86, 87, 98–100]. Myocardial tissue of power lifters using large doses of androgens has been shown to be infiltrated with fibrous tissue and fat droplets [87]. As many androgen users engage in high-intensity resistance exercise training, which also can induce left ventricular hypertrophy, it is not clear whether the left ventricular hypertrophy reported in power lifters is a consequence of strength training or of androgen use [100]. The inconsistency of findings across reports reduces the strength of inferences.

There are several case reports of sudden death among power athletes who were abusing androgens [84, 86, 98, 104–109]. Many of the sudden deaths have been associated with myocardial infarction. Some of the myocardial infarctions were deemed nonthrombotic leading to speculation that androgens might induce coronary vasospasm [100]. These case reports are largely anecdotal and a causative relationship between androgen use and the risk of sudden death is far from established. In fact, other studies have reported that testosterone is a vasodilator that can inhibit calcium channels. Power athletes using androgens often have short QT intervals but increased QT dispersion in contrast to endurance athletes with similar LV mass who have long QT intervals but do not have increased QT dispersion [103]. QT interval dispersion has been used as a noninvasive marker of susceptibility to arrhythmias [110]; we do not know whether this predisposes power lifters who abuse large doses of androgens to ventricular arrhythmias.

Psychiatric and Behavioral Effects of Androgens in Athletes

Anecdotal reports of rage reaction in androgen users, referred to as "roid rage," have attracted a great deal of media attention. However, placebo-controlled trials of testosterone have shown inconsistent changes in anger scores or measures of aggressive behaviors [71, 111–115]. Several factors may have contributed to this inconsistency of results across trials. The instruments used to measure aggressive behavior have varied across trials, and it is possible that the self-reporting question-naires did not have sufficient sensitivity to detect small but significant changes in aggression. Differences in weight training and related practices, concurrent use of other substances such as alcohol, psychoactive drugs, and dietary supplements, and pre-existing personality or psychiatric disorders are important confounders in interpretation of data related to behavioral effects of androgens [5]. None of the controlled trials of testosterone has demonstrated significant change in aggression at physiologic replacement doses of testosterone. In fact, testosterone replacement in healthy androgen-deficient men has been reported to improve positive aspects of mood and attenuate negative aspects of mood [116]. It is notable that only a small number of subjects (less than 5%) in controlled trials have demonstrated marked increases in aggression measures, and only with the use of supraphysiologic doses of testosterone; a majority of participants show little or no change [6, 71, 111, 112, 114, 115]. It is possible that high doses of androgens might provoke rage reactions in a subset of individuals with pre-existing psychopathology. Indeed, aggressive individuals – perhaps those with certain personality disorders – may be more prone to abuse androgens. In one survey, more androgen users than controls had worked as doormen or bouncers [117]. Among certain groups of criminals, the risk of having been convicted of a weapons offense was higher for androgen users than for nonusers [118]. Anecdotal reports suggest that among individuals with prior histories of psychiatric disorders or antisocial personality disorder or violence, the use of high doses of androgens might predispose men to violent or homicidal behavior [119].

It is possible that because of strong societal constraints against aggressive behav-ior, the self-reporting instruments fail to capture changes in the participant's behavior. However, when confronted with a provocative challenge, the individuals receiving high doses of androgens might display unexpectedly high level of aggression and rage. This hypothesis was tested by Kouri et al. [114], who reported that administra-tion of supraphysiologic doses (600 mg weekly) of testosterone enanthate to healthy, young men was associated with a significant increase in aggressive responses than placebo administration. In this study, healthy young men received in random order either placebo or graded doses of testosterone [114]. The participants were asked to play a game against a fictitious opponent, although the participants were unaware that the opponent was fictitious. The participants received a financial reward if they pressed button A or they could take money away from a fictitious opponent (aggres-sive responding) by pressing button B [114]. The objective of the game was to win as much money as possible; an insightful individual would have recognized that the best strategy to achieve that goal was to keep on pressing button A. Remarkably, individuals receiving supraphysiologic doses (600 mg weekly) of testosterone enanthate opted to select button B (to punish the fictitious opponent) with greater frequency and thus had higher scores on aggressive responding than those associated with no testosterone or lower doses of testosterone [114]. Thus, when provoked by a hostile situation, the level of aggressive response was higher when individuals were receiving high doses of testosterone than when they were receiving placebo or lower doses of testosterone enanthate [114].

Mood disorders, such as mania, hypomania, or major depression are highly prevalent among androgen users [23, 120–122]. Major depression has been reported during periods of androgen use but is more often observed during withdrawal from high dose androgen use [23, 120, 121]. High frequency of hypomania and depression, rigid dietary practices, and dissatisfaction with their body image also has been reported in women using high doses of androgens [123].

Kanayama et al. [124] have reported a high frequency of prior androgen abuse among male substance abusers [124]. In a sample of 223 male substance abusers, who were hospitalized for the treatment of alcohol, cocaine, and opioid dependence, 13% reported prior androgen use, leading Kanayama et al. [124] to speculate that androgen abuse may predispose some individuals to substance abuse.

Liver Toxicity

Liver abnormalities are uncommon in individuals using parenteral testosterone or its esters; however, the elevations of liver enzymes, cholestatic jaundice, hepatic neoplasms, and peliosis hepatis have been reported mostly with the use of oral, 17-alpha alkylated androgens [74, 75, 125–129]. Most case reports of hepatic neoplasms in association with androgen use have been reported in patients with myelodysplastic syndromes [130]. It is not clear whether elevations in AST and ALT during androgen administrations are the result of liver dysfunction or of muscle injury resulting from strength training or a direct transcriptional effect of androgens on AST gene [75, 76]. However, AST and ALT elevations have been seen almost exclusively with orally administered androgens.

The Suppression of Hypothalamic–Pituitary–Testicular Axis

Through their expected negative feedback effect at the pituitary and hypothalamic level, androgens suppress pituitary LH and FSH secretion and thereby inhibit endogenous testosterone production and spermatogenesis [131, 132]. Androgens, alone or in combination with GnRH analogs or progestins are being investigated as potential male contraceptives (Handelsman, 1995 #808). Therefore, men using androgens may experience subfertility or infertility [133].

The long-term suppression of the hypothalamic–pituitary–testicular axis is a serious complication of androgen use that may increase the risk of continued androgen use. The recovery of the hypothalamic–pituitary axis after discontinuation of androgen use may take varying length of time ranging from weeks to months. The speed of recovery may vary with the dose and duration of prior androgen use [134–137]. Upon cessation of exogenous androgen use, circulating testosterone concentrations fall to very low levels resulting in symptoms of severe androgen deficiency, including loss of sexual desire and function, depressed mood, and hot flushes. These symptoms may persist until the endogenous axis recovers, and may be so bothersome to some individuals that they may revert back to using androgens or seek other psychoactive drugs. Anecdotally, aromatase inhibitors and hCG have been used based on the belief that these drugs can accelerate the recovery of the hypothalamic–pituitary–testicular axis, although there is no evidence to support this premise. Thus, the prolonged suppression of hypothalamic–pituitary–testicular axis can perpetuate the vicious cycle of androgen abuse followed by symptomatic androgen deficiency during withdrawal, leading to continued use and dependence [135–137].

Gynecomastia

Breast tenderness and breast enlargement are common among androgen users [21, 24, 138], affecting almost half of the androgen users. In one series of 63 patients referred for surgical correction of gynecomastia, 20 men had used anabolic steroids [138]. Athletes often use an aromatase inhibitor or an estrogen antagonist in combination with androgens to prevent breast enlargement.

Androgen Abuse and Insulin Resistance

The effects of testosterone on insulin sensitivity have been inconsistent across trials and depend on the dose and the type of androgen used. In cross-sectional studies, low testosterone levels have been associated with increased risk of insulin resistance and type 2 diabetes mellitus, although it is not clear whether this represents an androgen effect or SHBG effect [139]. Holmang et al. reported that lowering of testosterone levels in male rats induces insulin resistance; testosterone replacement of castrated rats improves measures of insulin sensitivity [140]. However, supraphysiologic doses of testosterone impair insulin sensitivity [140]. Orally administered androgens also have been associated with insulin resistance, glucose intolerance, and diabetes mellitus [141, 142].

Risks Associated with Intramuscular Injections of Androgens

A significant fraction of those who administer androgens by intramuscular injections use unsafe injection practices [24] thus increasing the risk of local and systemic infections, and sepsis [22]. Additionally, needle sharing and the use of improperly sterilized needles and syringes render these individuals susceptible to hepatitis, HIV, or other blood-borne pathogens.

Risks Associated with Excessive Muscle Hypertrophy

Androgen use may result in excessive muscle hypertrophy without compensatory adaptations in the associated tendons, ligaments, and joints. These dissociated changes in muscle may predispose athletes using androgens to the risk of tendon injury and rupture, and joint disorders [143].

Polysubstance Abuse Among Androgen Abusers

The use of multiple drugs is common among androgen users; for instance, in some surveys 90% of androgen users also abused other drugs, including stimulants like amphetamine and cocaine [21, 24] and almost a quarter of androgen users took growth hormone or insulin [24]. Other drugs of abuse may include alcohol, cannabis, cocaine, amphetamine, heroin, and ephedra; some of these drugs may be associated with potentially even more serious medical complications than androgens. Recent reports suggest that androgen use is growing among users of other drugs to counteract the anorexia and weight loss associated with the use of street drugs [144].

Other Concerns

There are concerns about potential effects of androgens on the risk of prostate disease [2, 3, 145]. The long-term effects of supraphysiologic doses of androgens on the risk of prostate cancer, benign prostatic hypertrophy, and lower urinary tract symptoms are unknown.

Medical Issues Associated with Androgen Use Among Women

Women taking androgens may undergo masculinization and experience hirsutism, acne, deepening of voice, enlargement of clitoris, widening of upper torso, decreased breast size, menstrual irregularities, and male pattern baldness [128, 146]. Some of these adverse effects may not be reversible. In addition, epidemiologic studies have reported an association of elevated testosterone concentrations in women with increased risk of insulin resistance and diabetes mellitus [147].

Medical Issues Associated with Androgen Use Among Children

In addition to the adverse effects observed in adults, children may be susceptible to some unique adverse effects of androgens [148–150]. Pre or peripubertal boys and girls may undergo premature epiphyseal fusion, which may result in reduced adult height [148, 150]. Androgen abuse by children is associated with other unhealthy behaviors, such as the use of alcohol, tobacco and other drugs, less frequent seat belt use, more sexual activity, antisocial behavior, declining academic performance, and more fasting, vomiting, diet pill, and laxative use by young girls [150]. Boys may undergo premature pubertal changes while girls may experience virilization.

Hormone Precursors

Delta-4-Androstenedione

Although the Anabolic Steroid Control Act passed by the US Congress in 1990 had banned the sale and nonmedical use of androgens, the Dietary Supplement and Health Education Act of 1994 allowed the over-the-counter sales of androgen precursors, such as delta-4-androstenedione and dehydroepiandrosterone (DHEA) as dietary supplements. Mark Maguire's public admission of the use of delta-4-androstenedione during a summer of spectacular home runs unleashed explosive growth in the use and sales of these androgen precursors. Produced primarily by the gonads and the adrenal glands, androstenedione can be converted to testosterone by 17-β-hydroxysteroid dehydrogenase as well as to estrone by CYP19aromatase. Because it is a precursor to testosterone, exogenous administration of delta-4-androstenedione could potentially increase serum testosterone levels and produce the desired ergogenic effects. Some studies that used relatively low doses of androstenedione failed to demonstrate significant increments in serum testosterone levels or gains in lean body mass [28, 29]. However, Jasuja et al. [30] demonstrated conclusively that delta-4-androstenedione binds to androgen receptor, albeit with substantially lower affinity than dihydrotestosterone, causes nuclear translocation of the androgen receptor, and promotes myogenic differentiation. The effects of 4-androstenedione on myogenesis were inhibited by bicalutamide, an AR-antagonist. Moreover, supraphysiologic doses of androstenedione (500 mg given three times daily for a total daily dose of 1,500 mg) administered to hypogonadal men resulted in increased levels of serum androstenedione, total and free testosterone, estradiol and estrone, and was associated with significant gains in fat-free mass and muscle strength [30]. These data demonstrated unequivocally that delta-4-androstenedione is a bona fide androgen, albeit a weak one, which, when administered in sufficiently high doses, exerts significant anabolic effects.

The long-term effects of androstenedione on health are unknown. Because it is an androgen, it can result in unfavorable changes in lipid profile such as decreased HDL cholesterol levels and alter low-density lipoprotein (LDL)/HDL ratio. Increases in serum estrogen concentrations may potentially cause gynecomastia and infertility. Elevations in testosterone levels may cause acne and potentially increase the risk of prostate diseases.

Dehydroepiandrosterone

DHEA, an androgen precursor, and its sulfated form (DHEA-S) are the most abundant circulating adrenal steroids and are produced primarily in the adrenal glands. DHEA acts directly on the androgen receptor or indirectly via its conversion to testosterone, estrone and estradiol. Men have significantly higher levels of DHEA and DHEA-S than women; the DHEA levels peak in early adulthood and decline progressively with age. Although DHEA is a weak androgen, it is sold over the counter as a dietary health supplement and is marketed for its presumed anti-aging and anti-obesity properties.

Being a precursor to testosterone, DHEA has been touted as an ergogenic drug. However, DHEA ingestion has not been proven to enhance serum testosterone levels. Nestler et al. revealed that serum testosterone levels were not increased even with DHEA doses as high as 1,600 mg/day [31]. The effects of DHEA supplementation on body composition and muscle strength have been inconsistent across trials. In a placebo-controlled randomized clinical trial, DHEA supplementation in elderly men and women had no beneficial effects on body composition, physical performance, insulin sensitivity, or quality of life [32], while another trial reported a decrease in fat mass [31]. There was also no additional benefit of DHEA administration on physical performance, body composition, and insulin sensitivity in postmenopausal women [33].

Clinical trials of DHEA in a variety of disease states, such as Alzheimer's [34], adrenal insufficiency [1], and systemic lupus erythematoses (SLE) [1] have been inconclusive. In one study, administration of 50 mg DHEA daily for 16 weeks in women with primary or secondary adrenal insufficiency was associated with improvements in scores for anxiety, depression, and sexual function but no significant changes were appreciated in body composition while other trials of DHEA supplementation in women with adrenal insufficiency failed to confirm the beneficial effects of DHEA on mood, well being or sexual function [1]. DHEA supplementation may have potential beneficial results in elderly patients with osteoporosis as several studies have noted improvement in bone mineral density with DHEA administration [35, 36].

Because neither the benefits nor the safety of DHEA supplementation has been demonstrated, its clinical use in any condition is not justified at present time. In 2004, the US Congress passed an amended version of the Anabolic Steroid Control Act that modified the definition of androgens and banned 26 additional compounds including prohormones such as androstenedione and DHEA.

Designer Androgens

The appearance of "designer androgens" that were developed solely for abuse while escaping detection through current screening and detection methods is a remarkably sinister development in sports. Several androgens or androgen precursors such as norbolethone (first discovered in 2002), tetrahydrogestrinone (THG) (2003), and desoxymethyltestosterone (DMT) (2005) were synthesized solely for abuse. These compounds have not undergone safety testing in animals or humans and pose unknown health risks. THG was synthesized by chemists at BALCO, Inc and sold to many elite athletes, including a number of Olympians and well-known baseball players. Its use escaped detection for many years because this compound was not on the list of banned substances and was not being tested. Fortuitously, a syringe containing residual amounts of THG was sent anonymously to US Antidoping Agency (USADA). Subsequent studies established THG as a potent androgen in vitro and in vivo [151].

Since the first report in the late-1990s, the field of selective androgen receptor modulators (SARMs) has grown tremendously. SARMs act as full agonist in the skeletal muscle and bone while only as partial agonist in prostate tissue. The first generation SARMS are being developed as function promoting therapies for functional limitations associated with aging and chronic illness or for osteoporosis. The initial human trials of the first generation SARMs have shown small increments in fat-free mass. However, recognizing their potential for abuse, in early 2008, WADA prohibited the use of SARMs in sports.

References

1. Wilson JD. Androgen abuse by athletes. Endocr Rev. 1988; 9:181–199.
2. Bhasin S, Calof O, Storer TW, et al. Drug insights: anabolic applications of testosterone and selective androgen receptor modulators in aging and chronic illness. Nat Clin Pract Endocrinol Metab. 2006; 2:133–140.
3. Bhasin S, Cunningham GR, Hayes FJ, Matsumoto AM, Snyder PJ, Swerdloff RS, Montori VM. Testosterone therapy in adult men with androgen deficiency syndromes: an endocrine society clinical practice guideline. J Clin Endocrinol Metab. 2006; 91:1995–2010.
4. Yesalis CE, III, Bahrke MS, Kopstein AN, Baruskiewicz CK. Incidence onabolic steroid use: a discussion of methodological issues. In: Yesalis CE, III ed. 2000. Anabolic steroids in sports and exercise, Second ed. Champaign, IL: Human Kinetics; 73–115.

5. Yesalis CE, Barsukiewicz CK, Kopstein AN, Bahrke MS. Trends in anabolic-androgenic steroid use among adolescents. Arch Pediatr Adolesc Med. 1997; 151:1197–1206.
6. Yesalis CE, Kennedy NJ, Kopstein AN, Bahrke MS. Anabolic-androgenic steroid use in the United States. JAMA. 1993; 270:1217–1221.
7. Hoffman JR, Kraemer WJ, Bhasin S, Storer T, Ratamess NA, Haff GG, Willoughby DS, Rogol AD. Position stand on androgen and human growth hormone use. J Strength Cond Res/National Strength & Conditioning Association. 2009; 23:S1–S59.
8. Medicine ACoS. Position stand: the use of anabolic-androgenic steroids in sports. Med Sci Sports Exerc. 1987; 19:534–539.
9. Catlin DH, Fitch KD, Ljungqvist A. Medicine and science in the fight against doping in sport. J Intern Med. 2008; 264:99–114.
10. Kopera H. The history of anabolic steroids and a review of clinical experience with anabolic steroids. Acta Endocrinol Suppl (Copenh). 1985; 271:11–18.
11. McDuff DR, Baron D. Substance use in athletics: a sports psychiatry perspective. Clin Sports Med. 2005; 24:885–897, ix–x.
12. Noakes TD. Tainted glory – doping and athletic performance. N Engl J Med. 2004; 351:847–849.
13. Prendergast HM, Bannen T, Erickson TB, Honore KR. The toxic torch of the modern Olympic Games. Vet Hum Toxicol. 2003; 45:97–102.
14. Wadler GI. Drug use update. Med Clin North Am. 1994; 78:439–455.
15. Shackleton C. Steroid analysis and doping control 1960–1980: scientific developments and personal anecdotes. Steroids. 2009; 74:288–295.
16. Wade N. Anabolic steroids: doctors denounce them, but athletes aren't listening. Science. 1972; 176:1399–1403.
17. Yesalis CE, Courson SP, Wright JE. History of anabolic steroid use in sport and exercise. In: Yesalis CE ed. Anabolic steroids in sports and exercise. 2000. Champaign, IL: Human Kinetics; 51–72.
18. Yamaguchi R, Johnston LD, O'Malley PM. Relationship between student illicit drug use and school drug-testing policies. J Sch Health. 2003; 73:159–164.
19. Clifford PR, Edmundson E, Koch WR, Dodd BG. Discerning the epidemiology of drug use among a sample of college students. J Drug Educ. 1989; 19:209–223.
20. McCabe SE, Brower KJ, West BT, Nelson TF, Wechsler H. Trends in non-medical use of anabolic steroids by U.S. college students: results from four national surveys. Drug Alcohol Depend. 2007; 90:243–251.
21. Evans NA. Gym and tonic: a profile of 100 male steroid users. Br J Sports Med. 1997; 31:54–58.
22. Evans NA. Local complications of self administered anabolic steroid injections. Br J Sports Med. 1997; 31:349–350.
23. Pope HG, Jr., Katz DL. Psychiatric and medical effects of anabolic-androgenic steroid use. A controlled study of 160 athletes. Arch Gen Psychiatry. 1994; 51:375–382.
24. Parkinson AB, Evans NA. Anabolic androgenic steroids: a survey of 500 users. Med Sci Sports Exerc. 2006; 38:644–651.
25. Evans NA. Current concepts in anabolic-androgenic steroids. Am J Sports Med. 2004; 32:534–542.
26. Bhasin S, Storer TW, Berman N, Yarasheski KE, Clevenger B, Phillips J, Lee WP, Bunnell TJ, Casaburi R. Testosterone replacement increases fat-free mass and muscle size in hypogonadal men. J Clin Endocrinol Metab. 1997; 82:407–413.
27. Brodsky IG, Balagopal P, Nair KS. Effects of testosterone replacement on muscle mass and muscle protein synthesis in hypogonadal men – a clinical research center study. J Clin Endocrinol Metab. 1996; 81:3469–3475.
28. Wang C, Cunningham G, Dobs A, Iranmanesh A, Matsumoto AM, Snyder PJ, Weber T, Berman N, Hull L, Swerdloff RS. Long-term testosterone gel (AndroGel) treatment maintains beneficial effects on sexual function and mood, lean and fat mass, and bone mineral density in hypogonadal men. J Clin Endocrinol Metab. 2004; 89:2085–2098.

82   K. Choong et al.

29. Snyder PJ, Peachey H, Berlin JA, Hannoush P, Haddad G, Dlewati A, Santanna J, Loh L, Lenrow DA, Holmes JH, Kapoor SC, Atkinson LE, Strom BL. Effects of testosterone replacement in hypogonadal men. J Clin Endocrinol Metab. 2000; 85:2670–2677.
30. Steidle C, Schwartz S, Jacoby K, Sebree T, Smith T, Bachand R. AA2500 testosterone gel normalizes androgen levels in aging males with improvements in body composition and sexual function. J Clin Endocrinol Metab. 2003; 88:2673–2681.
31. Mauras N, Hayes V, Welch S, Rini A, Helgeson K, Dokler M, Veldhuis JD, Urban RJ. Testosterone deficiency in young men: marked alterations in whole body protein kinetics, strength, and adiposity. J Clin Endocrinol Metab. 1998; 83:1886–1892.
32. Bhasin S, Storer TW, Berman N, Callegari C, Clevenger B, Phillips J, Bunnell TJ, Tricker R, Shirazi A, Casaburi R. The effects of supraphysiologic doses of testosterone on muscle size and strength in normal men. N Engl J Med. 1996; 335:1–7.
33. Hartgens F, Kuipers H. Effects of androgenic-anabolic steroids in athletes. Sports Med. 2004; 34:513–554.
34. Bhasin S, Woodhouse L, Casaburi R, Singh AB, Bhasin D, Berman N, Chen X, Yarasheski KE, Magliano L, Dzekov C, Dzekov J, Bross R, Phillips J, Sinha-Hikim I, Shen R, Storer TW. Testosterone dose-response relationships in healthy young men. Am J Physiol Endocrinol Metab. 2001; 281:E1172–E1181.
35. Woodhouse LJ, Reisz-Porszasz S, Javanbakht M, Storer TW, Lee M, Zerounian H, Bhasin S. Development of models to predict anabolic response to testosterone administration in healthy young men. Am J Physiol Endocrinol Metab. 2003; 284:E1009–E1017.
36. Bhasin S, Storer TW, Javanbakht M, Berman N, Yarasheski KE, Phillips J, Dike M, Sinha-Hikim I, Shen R, Hays RD, Beall G. Testosterone replacement and resistance exercise in HIV-infected men with weight loss and low testosterone levels. JAMA. 2000; 283:763–770.
37. Grinspoon S, Corcoran C, Askari H, Schoenfeld D, Wolf L, Burrows B, Walsh M, Hayden D, Parlman K, Anderson E, Basgoz N, Klibanski A. Effects of androgen administration in men with the AIDS wasting syndrome. A randomized, double-blind, placebo-controlled trial. Ann Intern Med. 1998; 129:18–26.
38. Grinspoon S, Corcoran C, Stanley T, Katznelson L, Klibanski A. Effects of androgen administration on the growth hormone-insulin-like growth factor I axis in men with acquired immunodeficiency syndrome wasting. J Clin Endocrinol Metab. 1998; 83:4251–4256.
39. Casaburi R, Bhasin S, Cosentino L, Porszasz J, Somfay A, Lewis MI, Fournier M, Storer TW. Effects of testosterone and resistance training in men with chronic obstructive pulmonary disease. Am J Respir Crit Care Med. 2004; 170:870–878.
40. Snyder PJ, Peachey H, Hannoush P, Berlin JA, Loh L, Lenrow DA, Holmes JH, Dlewati A, Santanna J, Rosen CJ, Strom BL. Effect of testosterone treatment on body composition and muscle strength in men over 65 years of age. J Clin Endocrinol Metab. 1999; 84:2647–2653.
41. Page ST, Amory JK, Bowman FD, Anawalt BD, Matsumoto AM, Bremner WJ, Tenover JL. Exogenous testosterone (T) alone or with finasteride increases physical performance, grip strength, and lean body mass in older men with low serum T. J Clin Endocrinol Metab. 2004; 90(3):1502–1510.
42. Kenny AM, Prestwood KM, Gruman CA, Marcello KM, Raisz LG. Effects of transdermal testosterone on bone and muscle in older men with low bioavailable testosterone levels. J Gerontol A Biol Sci Med Sci. 2001; 56:M266–M272.
43. Storer TW, Magliano L, Woodhouse L, Lee ML, Dzekov C, Dzekov J, Casaburi R, Bhasin S. Testosterone dose-dependently increases maximal voluntary strength and leg power, but does not affect fatigability or specific tension. J Clin Endocrinol Metab. 2003; 88:1478–1485.
44. Coviello AD, Kaplan B, Lakshman KM, Chen T, Singh AB, Bhasin S. Effects of graded doses of testosterone on erythropoiesis in healthy young and older men. J Clin Endocrinol Metab. 2008; 93:914–919.
45. Blanco CE, Popper P, Micevych P. Anabolic-androgenic steroid induced alterations in choline acetyltransferase messenger RNA levels of spinal cord motoneurons in the male rat. Neuroscience. 1997; 78:873–882.

46. Blanco CE, Zhan WZ, Fang YH, Sieck GC. Exogenous testosterone treatment decreases diaphragm neuromuscular transmission failure in male rats. J Appl Physiol. 2001; 90:850–856.

47. Leslie M, Forger NG, Breedlove SM. Sexual dimorphism and androgen effects on spinal motoneurons innervating the rat flexor digitorum brevis. Brain Res. 1991; 561:269–273.

48. Sinha-Hikim I, Artaza J, Woodhouse L, Gonzalez-Cadavid N, Singh AB, Lee MI, Storer TW, Casaburi R, Shen R, Bhasin S. Testosterone-induced increase in muscle size in healthy young men is associated with muscle fiber hypertrophy. Am J Physiol Endocrinol Metab. 2002; 283:E154–E164.

49. Kadi F. Cellular and molecular mechanisms responsible for the action of testosterone on human skeletal muscle. A basis for illegal performance enhancement. Br J Pharmacol. 2008; 154:522–528.

50. Kadi F, Bonnerud P, Eriksson A, Thornell LE. The expression of androgen receptors in human neck and limb muscles: effects of training and self-administration of androgenic-anabolic steroids. Histochem Cell Biol. 2000; 113:25–29.

51. Sinha-Hikim I, Roth SM, Lee MI, Bhasin S. Testosterone-induced muscle hypertrophy is associated with an increase in satellite cell number in healthy, young men. Am J Physiol Endocrinol Metab. 2003; 285:E197–E205.

52. Sinha-Hikim I, Taylor WE, Gonzalez-Cadavid NF, Zheng W, Bhasin S. Androgen receptor in human skeletal muscle and cultured muscle satellite cells: up-regulation by androgen treatment. J Clin Endocrinol Metab. 2004; 89:5245–5255.

53. MacLean HE, Chiu WS, Ma C, McManus JF, Davey RA, Cameron R, Notini AJ, Zajac JD. A floxed allele of the androgen receptor gene causes hyperandrogenization in male mice. Physiol Genomics. 2008; 33:133–137.

54. Ophoff J, Van Proeyen K, Callewaert F, De Gendt K, De Bock K, Vanden Bosch A, Verhoeven G, Hespel P, Vanderschueren D. Androgen signaling in myocytes contributes to the maintenance of muscle mass and fiber type regulation but not to muscle strength or fatigue. Endocrinology. 2009; 150:3558–3566.

55. Singh R, Artaza JN, Taylor WE, Braga M, Yuan X, Gonzalez-Cadavid NF, Bhasin S. Testosterone inhibits adipogenic differentiation in 3T3-L1 cells: nuclear translocation of androgen receptor complex with beta-catenin and T-cell factor 4 may bypass canonical Wnt signaling to down-regulate adipogenic transcription factors. Endocrinology. 2006; 147:141–154.

56. Singh R, Artaza JN, Taylor WE, Gonzalez-Cadavid NF, Bhasin S. Androgens stimulate myogenic differentiation and inhibit adipogenesis in C3H 10T1/2 pluripotent cells through an androgen receptor-mediated pathway. Endocrinology. 2003; 144:5081–5088.

57. Singh R, Bhasin S, Braga M, Artaza JN, Pervin S, Taylor WE, Krishnan V, Sinha SK, Rajavashisth TB, Jasuja R. Regulation of myogenic differentiation by androgens: cross talk between androgen receptor/beta-catenin and follistatin/transforming growth factor-beta signaling pathways. Endocrinology. 2009; 150:1259–1268.

58. Jasuja R, Ulloor J, Yengo CM, Choong K, Istomin AY, Livesay DR, Jacobs DJ, Swerdloff RS, Miksovska J, Larsen RW, Bhasin S. Kinetic and thermodynamic characterization of dihydrotestosterone-induced conformational perturbations in androgen receptor ligand-binding domain. Mol Endocrinol. 2009; 23:1231–1241.

59. Kochakian CD, Cohn L, et al. Effect of testosterone propionate on nitrogen and chloride excretion and body weight of castrated rats during recovery from fasting. Am J Physiol. 1948; 155:272–277.

60. Kochakian CD, Costa G. The effect of testosterone propionate on the protein and carbohydrate metabolism in the depancreatized-castrated dog. Endocrinology. 1959; 65:298–309.

61. Urban RJ, Bodenburg YH, Gilkison C, Foxworth J, Coggan AR, Wolfe RR, Ferrando A. Testosterone administration to elderly men increases skeletal muscle strength and protein synthesis. Am J Physiol. 1995; 269:E820–E826.

62. Ferrando AA, Sheffield-Moore M, Paddon-Jones D, Wolfe RR, Urban RJ. Differential anabolic effects of testosterone and amino acid feeding in older men. J Clin Endocrinol Metab. 2003; 88:358–362.

63. Ferrando AA, Sheffield-Moore M, Yeckel CW, Gilkison C, Jiang J, Achacosa A, Lieberman SA, Tipton K, Wolfe RR, Urban RJ. Testosterone administration to older men improves muscle function: molecular and physiological mechanisms. Am J Physiol Endocrinol Metab. 2002; 282:E601–E607.

64. Choong K, Lakshman KM, Bhasin S. The physiological and pharmacological basis for the ergogenic effects of androgens in elite sports. Asian J Androl. 2008; 10:351–363.

65. Strauss RH, Liggett MT, Lanese RR. Anabolic steroid use and perceived effects in ten weight-trained women athletes. JAMA. 1985; 253:2871–2873.

66. Strauss RH, Yesalis CE. Anabolic steroids in the athlete. Annu Rev Med. 1991; 42:449–457.

67. Bahrke MS, Wright JE, Strauss RH, Catlin DH. Psychological moods and subjectively perceived behavioral and somatic changes accompanying anabolic-androgenic steroid use. Am J Sports Med. 1992; 20:717–724.

68. Bahrke MS, Wright JE, O'Connor JS, Strauss RH, Catlin DH. Selected psychological characteristics of anabolic-androgenic steroid users. N Engl J Med. 1990; 323:834–835.

69. Parssinen M, Kujala U, Vartiainen E, Sarna S, Seppala T. Increased premature mortality of competitive powerlifters suspected to have used anabolic agents. Int J Sports Med. 2000; 21:225–227.

70. Glazer G. Atherogenic effects of anabolic steroids on serum lipid levels. A literature review. Arch Intern Med. 1991; 151:1925–1933.

71. Daly RC, Su TP, Schmidt PJ, Pagliaro M, Pickar D, Rubinow DR. Neuroendocrine and behavioral effects of high-dose anabolic steroid administration in male normal volunteers. Psychoneuroendocrinology. 2003; 28:317–331.

72. Payne AH, Quinn PG, Rani CS. Regulation of microsome cytochrome P-450 enzymes and testosterone production in Leydig cells. Recent Prog Horm Res. 1985; 41:153–197.

73. Ansell JE, Tiarks C, Fairchild VK. Coagulation abnormalities associated with the use of anabolic steroids. Am Heart J. 1993; 125:367–371.

74. Soe KL, Soe M, Gluud C. Liver pathology associated with the use of anabolic-androgenic steroids. Liver. 1992; 12:73–79.

75. Dickerman RD, Pertusi RM, Zachariah NY, Dufour DR, McConathy WJ. Anabolic steroid-induced hepatotoxicity: is it overstated? Clin J Sport Med. 1999; 9:34–39.

76. Pertusi R, Dickerman RD, McConathy WJ. Evaluation of aminotransferase elevations in a bodybuilder using anabolic steroids: hepatitis or rhabdomyolysis? J Am Osteopath Assoc. 2001; 101:391–394.

77. Green GA, Uryasz FD, Petr TA, Bray CD. NCAA study of substance use and abuse habits of college student-athletes. Clin J Sport Med. 2001; 11:51–56.

78. Petersson A, Garle M, Holmgren P, Druid H, Krantz P, Thiblin I. Toxicological findings and manner of death in autopsied users of anabolic androgenic steroids. Drug Alcohol Depend. 2006; 81:241–249.

79. Petersson A, Garle M, Granath F, Thiblin I. Morbidity and mortality in patients testing positively for the presence of anabolic androgenic steroids in connection with receiving medical care. A controlled retrospective cohort study. Drug Alcohol Depend. 2006; 81:215–220.

80. Thiblin I, Lindquist O, Rajs J. Cause and manner of death among users of anabolic androgenic steroids. J Forensic Sci. 2000; 45:16–23.

81. Thiblin I, Runeson B, Rajs J. Anabolic androgenic steroids and suicide. Ann Clin Psychiatry. 1999; 11:223–231.

82. Melchert RB, Welder AA. Cardiovascular effects of androgenic-anabolic steroids. Med Sci Sports Exerc. 1995; 27:1252–1262.

83. Bonetti A, Tirelli F, Catapano A, Dazzi D, Dei Cas A, Solito F, Ceda G, Reverberi C, Monica C, Pipitone S, Elia G, Spattini M, Magnati G. Side effects of anabolic androgenic steroids abuse. Int J Sports Med. 2007; 29(8):679–687.

84. Dhar R, Stout CW, Link MS, Homoud MK, Weinstock J, Estes NA, III. Cardiovascular toxicities of performance-enhancing substances in sports. Mayo Clin Proc. 2005; 80:1307–1315.

85. Karila TA, Karjalainen JE, Mantysaari MJ, Viitasalo MT, Seppala TA. Anabolic androgenic steroids produce dose-dependant increase in left ventricular mass in power athletes, and this effect is potentiated by concomitant use of growth hormone. Int J Sports Med. 2003; 24:337–343.

86. Sullivan ML, Martinez CM, Gennis P, Gallagher EJ. The cardiac toxicity of anabolic steroids. Prog Cardiovas Dis. 1998; 41:1–15.
87. Nieminen MS, Ramo MP, Viitasalo M, Heikkila P, Karjalainen J, Mantysaari M, Heikkila J. Serious cardiovascular side effects of large doses of anabolic steroids in weight lifters. Eur Heart J. 1996; 17:1576–1583.
88. Maravelias C, Dona A, Stefanidou M, Spiliopoulou C. Adverse effects of anabolic steroids in athletes. A constant threat. Toxicol Lett. 2005; 158:167–175.
89. Basaria S, Nguyen T, Rosenson RS, Dobs AS. Effect of methyl testosterone administration on plasma viscosity in postmenopausal women. Clin Endocrinol (Oxf). 2002; 57:209–214.
90. Braga-Basaria M, Muller DC, Carducci MA, Dobs AS, Basaria S. Lipoprotein profile in men with prostate cancer undergoing androgen deprivation therapy. Int J Impot Res. 2006; 18:494–498.
91. Dobs AS, Bachorik PS, Arver S, Meikle AW, Sanders SW, Caramelli KE, Mazer NA. Interrelationships among lipoprotein levels, sex hormones, anthropometric parameters, and age in hypogonadal men treated for 1 year with a permeation-enhanced testosterone transdermal system. J Clin Endocrinol Metab. 2001; 86:1026–1033.
92. Friedl KE. Reappraisal of the health risks associated with the use of high doses of oral and injectable androgenic steroids. NIDA Res Monogr. 1990; 102:142–177.
93. Friedl KE, Hannan CJ, Jr., Jones RE, Plymate SR. High-density lipoprotein cholesterol is not decreased if an aromatizable androgen is administered. Metabolism. 1990; 39:69–74.
94. Whitsel EA, Boyko EJ, Matsumoto AM, Anawalt BD, Siscovick DS. Intramuscular testosterone esters and plasma lipids in hypogonadal men: a meta-analysis. Am J Med. 2001; 111:261–269.
95. Isidori AM, Giannetta E, Greco EA, Gianfrilli D, Bonifacio V, Isidori A, Lenzi A, Fabbri A. Effects of testosterone on body composition, bone metabolism and serum lipid profile in middle-aged men: a meta-analysis. Clin Endocrinol (Oxf). 2005; 63:280–293.
96. Singh AB, Hsia S, Alaupovic P, Sinha-Hikim I, Woodhouse L, Buchanan TA, Shen R, Bross R, Berman N, Bhasin S. The effects of varying doses of T on insulin sensitivity, plasma lipids, apolipoproteins, and C-reactive protein in healthy young men. J Clin Endocrinol Metab. 2002; 87:136–143.
97. Jockenhovel F, Bullmann C, Schubert M, Vogel E, Reinhardt W, Reinwein D, Muller-Wieland D, Krone W. Influence of various modes of androgen substitution on serum lipids and lipoproteins in hypogonadal men. Metabolism. 1999; 48:590–596.
98. Dickerman RD, McConathy WJ, Schaller F, Zachariah NY. Cardiovascular complications and anabolic steroids. Eur Heart J. 1996; 17:1912.
99. Kennedy MC, Lawrence C. Anabolic steroid abuse and cardiac death. Med J Aust. 1993; 158:346–348.
100. Payne JR, Kotwinski PJ, Montgomery HE. Cardiac effects of anabolic steroids. Heart (British Cardiac Society). 2004; 90:473–475.
101. De Piccoli B, Giada F, Benettin A, Sartori F, Piccolo E. Anabolic steroid use in body builders: an echocardiographic study of left ventricle morphology and function. Int J Sports Med. 1991; 12:408–412.
102. Urhausen A, Albers T, Kindermann W. Are the cardiac effects of anabolic steroid abuse in strength athletes reversible? Heart (British Cardiac Society). 2004; 90:496–501.
103. Stolt A, Karila T, Viitasalo M, Mantysaari M, Kujala UM, Karjalainen J. QT interval and QT dispersion in endurance athletes and in power athletes using large doses of anabolic steroids. Am J Cardiol. 1999; 84:364–366, A369.
104. Hausmann R, Hammer S, Betz P. Performance enhancing drugs (doping agents) and sudden death – a case report and review of the literature. Int J Legal Med. 1998; 111:261–264.
105. Di Paolo M, Agozzino M, Toni C, Luciani AB, Molendini L, Scaglione M, Inzani F, Pasotti M, Buzzi F, Arbustini E. Sudden anabolic steroid abuse-related death in athletes. Int J Cardiol. 2007; 114:114–117.
106. Dickerman RD, Schaller F, Prather I, McConathy WJ. Sudden cardiac death in a 20-year-old bodybuilder using anabolic steroids. Cardiology. 1995; 86:172–173.

107. Fineschi V, Baroldi G, Monciotti F, Paglicci Reattelli L, Turillazzi E. Anabolic steroid abuse and cardiac sudden death: a pathologic study. Arch Pathol Lab Med. 2001; 125:253–255.
108. Fineschi V, Riezzo I, Centini F, Silingardi E, Licata M, Beduschi G, Karch SB. Sudden cardiac death during anabolic steroid abuse: morphologic and toxicologic findings in two fatal cases of bodybuilders. Int J Legal Med. 2007; 121:48–53.
109. Luke JL, Farb A, Virmani R, Sample RH. Sudden cardiac death during exercise in a weight lifter using anabolic androgenic steroids: pathological and toxicological findings. J Forensic Sci. 1990; 35:1441–1447.
110. Pye M, Quinn AC, Cobbe SM. QT interval dispersion: a non-invasive marker of susceptibility to arrhythmia in patients with sustained ventricular arrhythmias? Br Heart J. 1994; 71:511–514.
111. Tricker R, Casaburi R, Storer TW, Clevenger B, Berman N, Shirazi A, Bhasin S. The effects of supraphysiological doses of testosterone on angry behavior in healthy eugonadal men – a clinical research center study. J Clin Endocrinol Metab. 1996; 81:3754–3758.
112. Su TP, Pagliaro M, Schmidt PJ, Pickar D, Wolkowitz O, Rubinow DR. Neuropsychiatric effects of anabolic steroids in male normal volunteers. JAMA. 1993; 269:2760–2764.
113. Yates WR, Perry PJ, MacIndoe J, Holman T, Ellingrod V. Psychosexual effects of three doses of testosterone cycling in normal men. Biol Psychiatry. 1999; 45:254–260.
114. Kouri EM, Lukas SE, Pope HG, Jr., Oliva PS. Increased aggressive responding in male volunteers following the administration of gradually increasing doses of testosterone cypionate. Drug Alcohol Depend. 1995; 40:73–79.
115. Pope HG, Jr., Kouri EM, Hudson JI. Effects of supraphysiologic doses of testosterone on mood and aggression in normal men: a randomized controlled trial. Arch Gen Psychiatry. 2000; 57:133–140; discussion 155–136.
116. Wang C, Alexander G, Berman N, Salehian B, Davidson T, McDonald V, Steiner B, Hull L, Callegari C, Swerdloff RS. Testosterone replacement therapy improves mood in hypogonadal men – a clinical research center study. J Clin Endocrinol Metab. 1996; 81:3578–3583.
117. Midgley SJ, Heather N, Davies JB. Levels of aggression among a group of anabolic-androgenic steroid users. Med Sci Law. 2001; 41:309–314.
118. Klotz F, Garle M, Granath F, Thiblin I. Criminality among individuals testing positive for the presence of anabolic androgenic steroids. Arch Gen Psychiatry. 2006; 63:1274–1279.
119. Pope HG, Jr., Katz DL. Homicide and near-homicide by anabolic steroid users. J Clin Psychiatry. 1990; 51:28–31
120. Malone DA, Jr., Dimeff RJ, Lombardo JA, Sample RH. Psychiatric effects and psychoactive substance use in anabolic-androgenic steroid users. Clin J Sport Med. 1995; 5:25–31.
121. Uzych L. Anabolic-androgenic steroids and psychiatric-related effects: a review. Can J Psychiatry. 1992; 37:23–28.
122. Porcerelli JH, Sandler BA. Anabolic-androgenic steroid abuse and psychopathology. Psychiatr Clin North Am. 1998; 21:829–833.
123. Gruber A, Pope HG, Jr. Psychaitric and medical effects of anabolic-androgenic steroid use in women. Psychother Psychosom. 2000; 69:19–26.
124. Kanayama G, Cohane GH, Weiss RD, Pope HG. Past anabolic-androgenic steroid use among men admitted for substance abuse treatment: an underrecognized problem? J Clin Psychiatry. 2003; 64:156–160.
125. Cabasso A. Peliosis hepatis in a young adult bodybuilder. Med Sci Sports Exerc. 1994; 26:2–4.
126. Socas L, Zumbado M, Perez-Luzardo O, Ramos A, Perez C, Hernandez JR, Boada LD. Hepatocellular adenomas associated with anabolic androgenic steroid abuse in bodybuilders: a report of two cases and a review of the literature. Br J Sports Med. 2005; 39:e27.
127. Kosaka A, Takahashi H, Yajima Y, Tanaka M, Okamura K, Mizumoto R, Katsuta K. Hepatocellular carcinoma associated with anabolic steroid therapy: report of a case and review of the Japanese literature. J Gastroenterol. 1996; 31:450–454.
128. Pavlatos AM, Fultz O, Monberg MJ, Pharmd VA. Review of oxymetholone: a 17alpha-alkylated anabolic-androgenic steroid. Clin Ther. 2001; 23:789–801; discussion 771.
129. Calof O, Singh AB, Lee MJ, Urban RJ, Kenny AM, Tenover JL, Bhasin S. Adverse events associated with testosterone supplementation of older men. J Gerontol A Biol Sci Med Sci. 2005; 60:1451–1457.

130. Nakao A, Sakagami K, Nakata Y, Komazawa K, Amimoto T, Nakashima K, Isozaki H, Takakura N, Tanaka N. Multiple hepatic adenomas caused by long-term administration of androgenic steroids for aplastic anemia in association with familial adenomatous polyposis. J Gastroenterol. 2000; 35:557–562.
131. Gill GV. Anabolic steroid induced hypogonadism treated with human chorionic gonadotropin. Postgrad Med J. 1998; 74:45–46.
132. MacIndoe JH, Perry PJ, Yates WR, Holman TL, Ellingrod VL, Scott SD. Testosterone suppression of the HPT axis. J Investig Med. 1997; 45:441–447.
133. Lloyd FH, Powell P, Murdoch AP. Anabolic steroid abuse by body builders and male subfertility. BMJ. 1996; 313:100–101.
134. Jarow JP, Lipshultz LI. Anabolic steroid-induced hypogonadotropic hypogonadism. Am J Sports Med. 1990; 18:429–431.
135. Brower KJ. Anabolic steroid abuse and dependence. Curr Psychiatry Rep. 2002; 4:377–387.
136. Brower KJ, Blow FC, Young JP, Hill EM. Symptoms and correlates of anabolic-androgenic steroid dependence. Br J Addict. 1991; 86:759–768.
137. Brower KJ, Eliopulos GA, Blow FC, Catlin DH, Beresford TP. Evidence for physical and psychological dependence on anabolic androgenic steroids in eight weight lifters. Am J Psychiatry. 1990; 147:510–512.
138. Babigian A, Silverman RT. Management of gynecomastia due to use of anabolic steroids in bodybuilders. Plast Reconstr Surg. 2001; 107:240–242.
139. Ding EL, Song Y, Manson JE, Hunter DJ, Lee CC, Rifai N, Buring JE, Gaziano JM, Liu S. Sex hormone-binding globulin and risk of type 2 diabetes in women and men. N Engl J Med. 2009; 361(12): 1152–1163
140. Holmang A, Bjorntorp P. The effects of testosterone on insulin sensitivity in male rats. Acta Physiol Scand. 1992; 146:505–510.
141. Cohen JC, Hickman R. Insulin resistance and diminished glucose tolerance in powerlifters ingesting anabolic steroids. J Clin Endocrinol Metab. 1987; 64:960–963.
142. Wilson DM, Frane JW, Sherman B, Johanson AJ, Hintz RL, Rosenfeld RG. Carbohydrate and lipid metabolism in Turner syndrome: effect of therapy with growth hormone, oxandrolone, and a combination of both. J Pediatr. 1988; 112:210–217.
143. Evans NA, Bowrey DJ, Newman GR. Ultrastructural analysis of ruptured tendon from anabolic steroid users. Injury. 1998; 29:769–773.
144. Graham MR, Davies B, Grace FM, Kicman A, Baker JS. Anabolic steroid use: patterns of use and detection of doping. Sports Med. 2008; 38:505–525.
145. Bhasin S, Singh AB, Mac RP, Carter B, Lee MI, Cunningham GR. Managing the risks of prostate disease during testosterone replacement therapy in older men: recommendations for a standardized monitoring plan. J Androl. 2003; 24:299–311.
146. Derman RJ. Effects of sex steroids on women's health: implications for practitioners. Am J Med. 1995; 98:137S–143S.
147. Ding EL, Song Y, Malik VS, Liu S. Sex differences of endogenous sex hormones and risk of type 2 diabetes: a systematic review and meta-analysis. JAMA. 2006; 295:1288–1299.
148. Casavant MJ, Blake K, Griffith J, Yates A, Copley LM. Consequences of use of anabolic androgenic steroids. Pediatr Clin North Am. 2007; 54:677–690, x.
149. Rogol AD. Sex steroid and growth hormone supplementation to enhance performance in adolescent athletes. Curr Opin Pediatr. 2000; 12:382–387.
150. vandenBerg P, Neumark-Sztainer D, Cafri G, Wall M. Steroid use among adolescents: longitudinal findings from project EAT. Pediatrics. 2007; 119:476–486.
151. Jasuja R, Catlin DH, Miller A, Chang YC, Herbst KL, Starcevic B, Artaza JN, Singh R, Datta G, Sarkissian A, Chandsawangbhuwana C, Baker M, Bhasin S. Tetrahydrogestrinone is an androgenic steroid that stimulates androgen receptor-mediated, myogenic differentiation in C3H10T1/2 multipotent mesenchymal cells and promotes muscle accretion in orchidectomized male rats. Endocrinology. 2005; 146:4472–4478.

Chapter 10
Growth Hormone

Arthur Weltman

Introduction

Growth hormone (GH) is secreted by the anterior pituitary in a pulsatile pattern. Multiple GH isotypes and oligomers exist in plasma in addition to the predominant 22 kD protein [1–3]. Minor isoforms do not change uniquely in response to exercise. GH activates cells by dimerizing receptors and triggering a cascade of phosphorylation reactions that signal to the nucleus.

The amount of GH secreted in each pulse is under physiological control by peptidyl agonists and antagonists [4–7]. Brain (hypothalamic) GH-releasing hormone (GHRH) stimulates GH synthesis and secretion, and somatostatin (SS) inhibits GH release without affecting its synthesis [8, 9]. A GH-releasing peptide (GHRP), ghrelin, expressed in the stomach, anterior pituitary gland, and hypothalamus amplifies GH secretion via cognate receptor codistributed with the peptide [8–11]. These three effector molecules govern GH secretion by convergent mechanisms [12, 13]. Many of the metabolic effects of GH are mediated by insulin-like growth factor type I (IGF-I), which is synthesized in the liver and all nucleated cells under the control of GH and tissue-specific hormones [8].

GH secretion declines by approximately 14% per decade after age 40 [14–16] and is markedly reduced in obesity even in younger individuals [17, 18]. Whereas GH production falls by 50% every 7 years in men beginning in young adulthood [16, 18, 19], the decrease is nearly twofold less rapid in premenopausal women [20–23]. Many age-related physical adaptations resemble those recognized in GH-deficient adults, including reduced muscle mass and exercise capacity, increased body fat especially abdominal visceral fat, unfavorable lipid and lipoprotein profiles, reduction

A. Weltman (✉)
Department of Human Services, University of Virginia, Charlottesville, VA 22904, USA
and
Department of Medicine, University of Virginia, Charlottesville, VA 22904, USA
and
Exercise Physiology Program, University of Virginia, Charlottesville, VA 22904, USA
e-mail: alw2v@virginia.edu

E. Ghigo et al. (eds.), *Hormone Use and Abuse by Athletes*, Endocrine Updates 29,   89
DOI 10.1007/978-1-4419-7014-5_10, © Springer Science+Business Media, LLC 2011

in bone mineral density, and cerebro- and cardiovascular disease. Which is cause and which is effect is difficult to ascertain in that intraabdominal adiposity and limited exercise also predict reduced GH production [24, 25]. In most studies, administration of GH to GH-deficient adults and/or obese adults results in a reduction in body fat and visceral fat in particular, an increase in muscle mass and maximal oxygen consumption, and favorable changes in cardiometabolic risk profiles [26–30]. However, administration of GH to non-GHD young and older adults has resulted in equivocal findings [31–35].

The suggested benefits of GH relative to muscle mass increase and fat mass decrease coupled with the fact that GH is either not typically tested for in athletic settings or is currently difficult to detect makes GH an attractive drug for abuse by athletes. There are several recent reviews in the area of GH abuse in sports [36–40]. The present chapter will attempt to synthesize existing data related to GH administration in athletes and present probable scenarios related to new methods of GH abuse.

GH Abuse by Athletes

GH was suggested as a potential anabolic agent as early as 1983 by Dan Duchaine in his book "The Underground Steroid Handbook" [36, 41]. Two highly publicized cases of GH abuse in athletes were reported in 1988. The first involved the doping scandal during the Tour de France where a large quantity of GH found in one of the team support cars [38, 39] and the second involved the disqualification of Ben Johnson during the Summer Olympic games. Johnson ran the 100 m in 9.79 s and the eventual gold medal winner Carl Lewis ran 9.83 s (both times broke the existing world record). Although Johnson tested positive for steroids, he admitted under oath that he also abused GH [36, 38]. More disturbingly, a 1992 report indicated that ~5% of US high school students admitted to having taken GH and ~33% knew someone who had taken GH [42]. These students had little information about the potential side effects of GH use. As reviewed by Holt and Sonkson [39], a Chinese swimmer, Yuan Yuan, was stopped on entry into Perth (the site of the 1998 World Swimming Championships) with a suitcase full of GH that had been exported to China for therapy use. Several athletes have either admitted to, or been linked to, GH abuse, including Lyle Alzado (American Football player); Walter Reiterer (Australian Discus thrower); Bjarne Riis (a Danish cyclist and former stage winner at the Tour de France); Ivan Basso, Jan Ullrich, and other Tour de France riders (as part of the Spanish doping scandal – a ring that allegedly supplied riders and other athletes with banned drugs, doping expertise, and performance-enhancing blood transfusions); Marion Jones and Tim Montgomery (track); and Barry Bonds, Alex Rodriguez, and Sammy Sosa (baseball).

Why Athletes Abuse GH

GH is a powerful metabolic hormone. It has both anabolic and lipolytic effects that athletes believe will enhance performance. Most of the information that athletes have based their beliefs on are either anecdotal or related to information that has been derived from GH-deficient individuals.

Anabolic Effects of GH Administration in GHD

GH causes nitrogen retention. GH promotes positive protein balance in skeletal muscle by increasing protein anabolism and possibly by decreasing protein catabolism [36, 37, 39]. There is a synergistic action between insulin, IGF-I, and GH in promoting protein synthesis (see Fig. 2 from [39]). When GH-deficient adults are treated with GH, a large number of beneficial anabolic outcomes have been observed, including increased muscle mass, increased muscle strength, increased maximal exercise performance, increased maximal oxygen consumption, increased left ventricular mass, increased stroke volume, and increased cardiac output (for a more complete review, see [36, 39]).

Lipolytic Effects of GH Administration in GHD

The lipolytic effects of GH are well established [36, 37, 39]. GH administration in humans results in a stimulation in lipolysis and an increase in FFA concentrations [43]. GH has both direct and indirect effects on lipolysis. It directly stimulates lipolysis through activation of adenylyl cyclase, cAMP-dependent protein kinase and phosphorylation, and hormone-sensitive lipase [44]. GH is also thought to stimulate lipolysis indirectly by increasing the ability of adipocytes to respond to catecholamines [43].

When GH is administered to GHD adults and/or adults with relative GH deficiency (e.g., obese and older adults), a consistent decrease in fat mass and in abdominal visceral fat in particular is observed [26, 27, 45].

However, although the data obtained from GH-deficient adults provide useful information regarding the effects of GH replacement, there are several confounding factors, including GHD adults typically having very low fitness and strength levels, which will allow for maximization of the effect of GH treatment; most GHD subjects having underlying pathology (e.g., pituitary tumor); and GH treatment oftentimes being combined with other hormone treatment in GHD adults. These limitations make it difficult to translate findings to improved performance in athletes.

Effects of GH Treatment in Healthy Adults

A number of studies on the effects of GH on a variety of outcome measures in healthy adults have included both single-dose and multiple-dose GH studies. Liu et al. [38] recently completed a systematic review of 44 randomized controlled trials that compared GH treatment to no GH treatment in healthy adults. Their review suggests that while GH administration may increase fat-free mass, strength and exercise performance did not improve with GH, and that edema and fatigue were more common in the GH-treated subjects [38]. The authors concluded that claims that GH improves athletic performance are not supported by the available scientific literature.

Single-Dose GH Studies

A limited number of studies have examined the acute effects of GH administration on exercise performance and other outcome measures in healthy adults. Single-dose administration of GH may elevate blood lactate, glycerol, and free fatty acid concentration [31, 32] and may impair [31] or have no effect on exercise performance [33]. Results from our laboratory indicate that time of exercise initiation after GH administration did not affect total work (kcal), perception of effort, HR, or the blood lactate response to exercise [33]. We did observe a reduction in steady-state oxygen consumption during constant load exercise, which suggests that GH administration may result in greater economy [33].

GH Treatment Studies

Although there are several studies that have examined the effects of GH treatment on outcome measures related to athletic performance in healthy adults, most are short-term studies (e.g., treatment of less than 30 days). The majority of studies indicate that GH treatment reduces fat mass, and increases fat-free (or lean body) mass as also the basal metabolic rate (for a complete review, see [38]). However, it should be noted that fat-free mass includes both protein (e.g., muscle) and water, and as such it is possible that the increase in fat-free mass with GH administration may be due to an increase in total body water rather than an increase in muscle mass [46].

Yarasheski et al. [34, 35] examined the effects of GH administration on muscle strength and protein synthesis and reported that GH administration in combination with heavy resistance training did not affect strength or muscle protein synthesis above that observed with strength training alone. Similarly, GH treatment has little effect on exercise performance measures including cycling speed and power output obtained from maximal oxygen consumption [32, 46, 47].

Although the research on healthy adults is limited and GH treatment is short term, most investigators have concluded that GH administration has little effect on enhancing athletic performance. However, it should be realized that while the doses administered in the studies reviewed above were supraphysiological, they were likely less than the doses that abusing athletes take.

A world class athlete (Olympic gold and silver medalist) once told me that athletes usually discover what works (regardless whether it is legal or ethical) and suggested that "you scientists then tell us why it works after the fact." He is probably correct to a certain degree.

Athletes Doses of GH

Because GH is a banned substance, the doses that athletes use are difficult to evaluate. It has been suggested that athletes abusing GH take recombinant hGH three to four times per week at a dose of 10–25 IU/day to increase their lean body mass [48]. Furthermore, it is also likely that athletes use GH in combination with other doping agents (e.g., anabolic steroids and EPO). In power athletes, it is thought that GH is taken in 4–6 week cycles, similar to the pattern of steroid abuse, and that GH is likely stacked with steroid use [48]. Less is known about its use in endurance activities or about its use in combination with other doping agents designed to enhance endurance performance such as erythropoietin. Because athletes often use GH in combination with other performance-enhancing agents, it is difficult to assess the independent effects of GH on athletic performance in this setting. Although the effects of GH administration have not been impressive in controlled studies, anecdotal reports by competitive body builders suggest a dramatic increase in muscle size and strength after large doses of GH [48]. In addition, it is possible that the stimulating effect of GH on collagen synthesis may reduce the risk of injury to tendon and muscles, allowing for faster recovery from training and more frequent high-intensity workouts [37]. Based on the number of athletes who use and abuse this expensive drug, it is clear that athletes believe that GH, either alone or in combination with the cocktail of other drugs they are taking, provides them with a competitive edge.

Potential Adverse Effects of GH Abuse

The side effects of GH treatment in GH-deficient adults are well documented [49]. Common side effects include edema, arthralgias, and myalgias. About 10% of GHD adults treated with GH develop carpal tunnel syndrome. Less commonly reported side effects include atrial fibrillation, congestive heart failure, decreased insulin sensitivity, and cancer. It should be realized that these side effects occur with physiological replacement doses in GHD adults.

Athletes typically take pharmacological doses that are likely ten or more times greater than typical replacement doses. Although the long-term adverse effects of these megadoses are not known at present, some insights may be obtained from patients with acromegaly, a physiological condition of GH excess. Acromegalics have an increased risk of insulin resistance and diabetes (up to 40% become diabetic), hypertension, cardiomyopathy, and certain forms of cancer (colorectal, thyroid, breast, and prostate) [39]. It can be argued that long-term pharmacological abuse of GH by athletes will likely result in some of the adverse effects listed above. In addition, there are two other side effects that athletes should be aware of: (1) although all GH prescribed today is recombinant hGH, there is still GH available on the black market that comes from extracts of human pituitary glands. The reason pituitary-derived GH was withdrawn from the prescription market is that this is a source for Creutzfelt–Jacob disease, a disease characterized by slow progressive dementia [39]; (2) GH is administered via injection. Therefore, if syringes are not sterile or contaminated (e.g., shared), there is a risk of infections such as HIV/AIDS or hepatitis [48].

Detection of GH Abuse

Because of the apparent widespread abuse of GH in sports, a number of research groups have been working to develop tests to prove the administration of exogenous GH in athletes. Several different approaches have been used. The marker approach uses characteristic changes in end points of GH action (e.g., serum concentrations of IGF-I and markers of bone and soft tissue turnover), whereas the isoform approach detects changes in molecular isoform concentrations of GH caused by the administration of exogenous recombinant hGH [50]. Recently, high-sensitivity chemiluminescence immunoassays have been developed to preferentially detect phGH or rhGH for up to 36 h after a single injection of rhGH [51]. The most recent advances in detection of GH abuse are presented in much greater detail elsewhere in this update.

GH Secretagogues

GH secretagogues stimulate endogenous GH release [6, 8, 10, 11, 13]. A wide variety of secretagogues have been studied including hexarelin, GHRP-6, GHRP-2, GHRP-1, and MK0677. It has been suggested that the hypothalamic GH secretagogue receptor regulates GH secretion, feeding, and adiposity [11, 13]. The GH secretagogue receptor has also been isolated in nonhypothalamic areas of the brain, in the anterior pituitary, and in the stomach [13, 40]. In 1999, Kojima et al. discovered an endogenous stomach ligand and named this new hormone ghrelin [10]. We have reported that the administration of GHRP-2 may further enhance the stimulatory effect of exercise on GH secretion by opposing central actions of SS and/or by heightening endogenous GHRH release [52]. A number of drug companies are developing GH secretagogues for eventual market distribution. These drugs will have the potential to be subjected to abuse by athletes [40].

Gene Doping: The Next Frontier for Athletic Abuse

With recent advances in gene therapy, it is only a matter of time before this technique becomes available, to be abused by athletes [40]. Selective alteration of progrowth (IGF-I) and antigrowth (myostatin) factors will likely have much more powerful effects than the injection of rhGH [40].

Conclusions

It is clear that a substantial number of athletes resort to doping in order to obtain a competitive edge in sporting activities. The use of GH has become more common as athletes believe that it has both anabolic and lipolytic effects and that it is virtually undetectable during doping control testing. While much of the evidence regarding the effectiveness of GH administration has come from GH-deficient adults, controlled studies of GH treatment in healthy adults have not supported the claims that GH administration benefits athletic performance. However, it should be realized that abusing athletes tend to administer doses of GH that are much greater than the supraphysiological doses evaluated in healthy subjects and they often stack multiple doping agents. As such, it is difficult to evaluate the independent effects of GH use on athletic performance in these individuals. Notwithstanding the unethical nature of GH doping (which does not seem to faze many athletes), GH administration is associated with a variety of adverse effects. Although most are mild and reversible when physiological administration of GH is closely monitored by a supervising physician, there is concern about potential serious (e.g., life threatening) consequences of long-term use of megadoses of GH. Fortunately, detection techniques are improving, but athletes seem to find a way to beat the system in the short term. In the long term, many athletes are caught cheating and all athletes in their sport are tainted.

References

1. Baumann G. Growth hormone heterogeneity: genes, isohormones, variants and binding proteins. Endocr Rev. 1991; 12: 424–449.
2. Nindl BC, Kraemer WJ, Marx JO, et al. Growth hormone molecular heterogeneity and exercise. Exerc Sport Sci Rev. 2003; 31: 161–166.
3. Lewis UJ, Sinha YN, Lewis GP. Structure and properties of members of the hGH family: a review. Endocr J. 2000; 47(Suppl): S1–S8.

4. Arvat E, Ceda GP, Di Vito L, et al. Age-related variations in the neuroendocrine control, more than impaired receptor sensitivity, cause the reduction in the GH-releasing activity of GHRP's in human aging. Pituitary. 1998; 1: 51–58.
5. Mueller EE, Locatelli V, Cocchi D. Neuroendocrine control of growth hormone secretion. Physiol Rev. 1999; 79: 511–607.
6. Bowers CY. New insight into the control of growth hormone secretion. In: Kleinberg DL, Clemmons DR, eds. Central and Peripheral Mechanisms in Pituitary Disease. Bristal, UK: BioScientifica Ltd; 2002: 163–176.
7. Farhy LS, Straume M, Johnson ML, et al. A construct of interactive feedback control of the GH axis in the male. Am J Physiol. 2001; 281: R38–R51.
8. Giustina A, Veldhuis JD. Pathophysiology of the neuroregulation of growth hormone secretion in experimental animals and the human. Endocr Rev. 1998; 19(6): 717–797.
9. Hartman ML. Physiological regulators of growth hormone secretion. In: Juul A, Jorgensen JOL, eds. Growth Hormone in Adults. 2nd ed. Cambridge, UK: Cambridge University Press; 2000: 3–53.
10. Kojima M, Hiroshi H, Date Y, et al. Ghrelin is a growth-hormone releasing acylated peptide from stomach. Nature. 1999; 402: 656–666.
11. Shuto Y, Shibasaki T, Otagiri A, et al. Hypothalamic growth hormone secretagogue receptor regulates growth hormone secretion, feeding, and adiposity. J Clin Invest. 2002; 109: 1429–1436.
12. Veldhuis JD, Bowers CY. Three-peptide control of pulsatile and entropic feedback-sensitive modes of growth hormone secretion: modulation by estrogen and aromatizable androgen. J Pediatr Endocrinol. 2003; 16(Suppl. 3): 587–605.
13. Veldhuis JD, Bowers CY. Determinants of GH-releasing hormone and GH-releasing peptide synergy in men. Am J Physiol Endocrinol Metab. 2009; 296: E1085–E1092.
14. Rudman D, Kutner MH, Rogers CM, et al. Impaired growth hormone secretion in the adult population. J Clin Invest. 1981; 67: 1361–1369.
15. Zadik Z, Chalew SA, McCarter RJ, et al. The influence of age on the 24-hour integrated concentration of growth hormone in normal individuals. J Clin Endocrinol Metab. 1985; 60: 513–516.
16. Iranmanesh A, Lizarralde G, Veldhuis JD. Age and relative adiposity are specific negative determinants of the frequency and amplitude of growth hormone (GH) secretory bursts and the half-life of endogenous GH in healthy men. J Clin Endocrinol Metab. 1991; 73: 1081–1088.
17. Veldhuis JD, Iranmenesh A, Ho KKY, et al. Dual defects in pulsatile growth hormone secretion and clearance subserve the hyposomatotropism of obesity in man. J Clin Endocrinol Metab. 1991; 72: 51–59.
18. Veldhuis JD, Liem AY, South S, et al. Differential impact of age, sex steroid hormones, and obesity on basal versus pulsatile growth hormone secretion in men as assessed in an ultrasensitive chemiluminescence assay. J Clin Endocrinol Metab. 1995; 80: 3209–3222.
19. Iranmanesh A, South S, Liem AY, et al. Unequal impact of age, percentage body fat, and serum testosterone concentrations on the somatotrophic, IGF-I, and IGF-binding protein responses to a three-day intravenous growth hormone-releasing hormone pulsatile infusion in men. Eur J Endocrinol. 1998; 139: 59–71.
20. Asplin CM, Faria AC, Carlsen EC, et al. Alterations in the pulsatile mode of growth hormone release in men and women with insulin-dependent diabetes mellitus. J Clin Endocrinol Metab. 1989; 69: 239–245.
21. Winer LM, Shaw MA, Baumann G. Basal plasma growth hormone levels in man: new evidence for rhythmicity of growth hormone secretion. J Clin Endocrinol Metab. 1990; 70: 1678–1686.
22. Weltman A, Weltman JY, Hartman ML, et al. Relationship between age, percentage body fat, fitness, and 24-hour growth hormone release in healthy young adults: effects of gender. J Clin Endocrinol Metab. 1994; 78: 543–548.
23. van den Berg G, Veldhuis JD, Frolich M, et al. An amplitude-specific divergence in the pulsatile mode of GH secretion underlies the gender difference in mean GH concentrations in men and premenopausal women. J Clin Endocrinol Metab. 1996; 81: 2460–2466.

24. Clasey JL, Weltman A, Patrie J, et al. Abdominal visceral fat and fasting insulin are important predictors of 24-hour GH release independent of age, gender and other physiological factors. J Clin Endocrinol Metab. 2001; 86: 3845–3852.
25. Vahl N, Jorgensen JO, Skjaerback, C, et al. Abdominal adiposity rather than age and sex predicts the mass and patterned regularity of growth hormone secretion in mid-life healthy adults. Am J Physiol. 1997; 272: E1108–E1116.
26. Johannsson G, Marin P, Lonn L, et al. Growth hormone treatment of abdominally obese men reduces abdominal fat mass, improves glucose and lipoprotein metabolism, and reduces diastolic blood pressure. J Clin Endocrinol Metab. 1997; 82: 727–734.
27. Franco C, Brandberg J, Lonn L, et al. Growth hormone treatment reduces abdominal visceral fat in postmenopausal women with abdominal obesity: a 12-month placebo-controlled trial. J Clin Endocrinol Metab. 2005; 90: 1466–1474.
28. Colao A, di Somma C, Cuocolo A, et al. Improved cardiovascular risk factors and cardiac performance after 12 months of growth hormone (GH) replacement in young adult patients with GHD. J Clin Endocrinol Metab. 2001; 86: 1874–1881.
29. Johannsson G, Grimby G, Sunnerhagen KS, et al. Two years of growth hormone (GH) treatment increase isometric and isokinetic muscle strength in GH-deficient adults. J Clin Endocrinol Metab. 1997; 82: 2877–2884.
30. Hartman, ML, Weltman A, Zagar A, et al. Growth hormone replacement therapy in adults with growth hormone deficiency improves maximal oxygen consumption (VO_2 max) independently of dosing regimen or physical activity. J Clin Endocrinol Metab. 2008; 93: 125–130.
31. Lange KH, Larsson B, Flyvbjerg A, et al. Acute growth hormone administration causes exaggerated increases in plasma lactate and glycerol during moderate to high intensity bicycling in trained young men. J Clin Endocrinol Metab. 2002; 87: 4966–4975.
32. Healy ML, Gibney J, Pentecost C, et al. Effects of high-dose growth hormone on glucose and glycerol metabolism at rest and during exercise in endurance-trained athletes. J Clin Endocrinol Metab. 2006; 91: 320–327.
33. Irving BA, Patrie JT, Anderson SM, et al. The effects of time following acute growth hormone administration on metabolic and power output measurements during acute exercise. J Clin Endocrinol Metab. 2004; 89: 4298–4305.
34. Yarasheski KE, Campbell JA, Smith K, et al. Effect of growth hormone and resistance exercise on muscle growth in young men. Am J Physiol. 1992; 262: E261–E267.
35. Yarasheski KE, Zachweija JJ, Angelopoulous TJ, et al. Short term growth hormone treatment does not increase muscle protein synthesis in experienced weight lifters. J Appl Physiol. 1993; 74: 3073–3076.
36. Gibney J, Healy ML, Sonkson PH. The growth hormone/insulin-like growth factor-I axis in exercise and sport. Endocr Rev. 2007; 28: 608–624.
37. Ehrnborg C, Rosen T. Physiological and pharmacological basis for the ergogenic effects of growth hormone in elite sports. Asian J Androl. 2008; 10: 373–383.
38. Liu H, Bravata DM, Olkin I, et al. Systematic review: the effects of growth hormone on athletic performance. Ann Intern Med. 2008; 148: 747–758.
39. Holt RIG, Sonkson PH. Growth hormone, IGF-I and insulin and their abuse in sport. Br J Pharmacol. 2008; 154: 542–556.
40. Jordi S, Gutierrez-Gallego R, Ventura R, et al. Growth hormone in sport: beyond Beijing 2008. Ther Drug Monit. 2009; 31: 3–12.
41. Duchaine D. Underground Steroid Handbook. Venice, CA: HLR Technical Books; 1983.
42. Rickert VI, Pawlak-Morello C, Sheppard V, et al. Human growth hormone: a new substance of abuse among adolescents? Clin Pediatr. 1992; 31: 723–726.
43. Hanson TK. Pharmacokinetics and acute lipolytic actions of growth hormone: impact of age, body composition, binding proteins, and other hormones. Growth Horm IGF Res. 2002; 12: 342–358.
44. Yip RG, Goldman HM. Growth hormone and dexamethasone stimulate lipolysis and activate cyclase in rat adipocytes by selectively shifting Gi α2 to lower density membrane fractions. Endocrinology. 1999; 140: 1219–1227.

45. Bengtsson BA, Eden S, Lonn L, et al. Treatment of adults with growth hormone (GH) deficiency with recombinant GH. J Clin Endocrinol Metab. 1993; 76: 309–317.
46. Ehrnborg C, Ellegard L, Bosaeus I, et al. Supraphsyiological growth hormone: less fat, more extra-cellular fluid but uncertain effects on muscles in healthy, active young adults. Clin Endocrinol. 2005; 62: 449–467.
47. Berggren A, Ehrnborg, C, Rosen T, et al. Short-term administration of supraphysiological recombinant human GH (growth hormone) does not increase maximum endurance exercise capacity in healthy, active young men and women with normal GH-insulin-like growth factor I axes. J Clin Endocrinol Metab. 2005; 90: 3268–3273.
48. Saugy M, Robinson N, Saudan C, et al. Human growth hormone doping in sport. Br J Sports Med. 2006; 40: i35–i39.
49. Guistina A, Barkan A, Chanson P, et al. Guidelines for the treatment of growth hormone excess and growth hormone deficiency is adults. J Endocrinol Invest. 2008; 31: 820–838.
50. Bidlingmaier M, Strausburger CJ. Technology insight: detecting growth hormone abuse in athletes. Nat Clin Pract Endocrinol Metab. 2007; 3: 769–777.
51. Bidlingmaier M, Suhr J, Ernst A, et al. High-sensitivity chemiluminescence immunoassays for detection of growth hormone doping in sports. Clin Chem. 2009; 55: 445–453.
52. Wideman L, Weltman JY, Patrie JT, et al. Synergy of L-arginine and GHRP-2 stimulation of growth hormone in men and women: modulation by exercise. Am J Physiol Regul Integr Comp Physiol. 2000; 279: R1467–R1477.

Chapter 11
Erythropoietin

Wolfgang Jelkmann

Introduction

Erythropoietin (Epo), a hormone predominantly produced in the kidneys, is an essential growth factor for the erythrocytic progenitors in the bone marrow. Tissue hypoxia is the physiological stimulus for *Epo* expression and erythropoiesis. The production of red blood cells (RBC; normally $2–3 \times 10^{11}$ per day) may severalfold increase on hypoxic stress. Recombinant human Epo (rhEpo) has been clinically used for treatment of the anemia of chronic kidney disease (CKD) for two decades [1]. rhEpo and second generation erythropoiesis-stimulating agents (ESAs) such as the rhEpo analog Darbepoetin alfa and the Epo-mimetic peptide Hematide™ are included in the list of prohibited substances in sports by the World Anti-Doping Agency (www.wada-ama.org). ESAs exert ergogenic effects by increasing RBC and hemoglobin (Hb) mass, and thereby the aerobic capacity (VO_{2max}) [2], which depends on the difference between the arterial and venous O_2 content, and the maximal cardiac output. Since the arterial O_2 saturation is almost 100% in healthy persons at sea level, the arterial O_2 content hinges mainly on the Hb concentration ("O_2 capacity": about 1.34 ml O_2/g Hb). This article reviews the physiological role of Epo in RBC production, the various ESAs developed for clinical use, and the methods for their detection if misused in sports.

W. Jelkmann (✉)
Institute of Physiology, University of Luebeck, Ratzeburger Allee 160,
D-23538 Luebeck, Germany
e-mail: jelkmann@physio.uni-luebeck.de

E. Ghigo et al. (eds.), *Hormone Use and Abuse by Athletes*, Endocrine Updates 29,
DOI 10.1007/978-1-4419-7014-5_11, © Springer Science+Business Media, LLC 2011

Physiology of Epo

Structure of Epo

Epo is a 30 kDa glycoprotein of 165 amino acids and 40% carbohydrate. It possesses 3 tetraantennary N-linked (at Asn^{24}, Asn^{38} and Asn^{83}) and 1 small O-linked (at Ser^{126}) acidic glycans. The N-glycans are critical for Epo's secretion, molecular stability, receptor (Epo-R) binding, and in vivo bioactivity. Both endogenous Epo and rhEpo exhibit several glycosylation isoforms, which can be distinguished by isoelectric focusing (IEF) or electrophoresis followed by immunoblotting, or by high performance liquid chromatography [3, 4]. The structure of the glycan isoforms of rhEpo preparations depends greatly on the culturing conditions of the *Epo*-transfected cells and the purification procedures of the products [5].

Erythropoietic Action of Epo

Epo binds to specific homodimeric receptors (Epo-R) in the membrane of the erythrocytic progenitors. The human Epo-R monomer is a 484 amino acids glycoprotein belonging to the cytokine class I-receptor superfamily [6]. On binding of one Epo molecule, the Epo-R dimer undergoes a conformational change which results in the activation of cytosolic Janus kinases 2 (JAK2) and, in sequence, other signal transducing enzymes and transcription factors [7]. Epo suppresses the programmed cell death ("apoptosis") of the colony-forming units-erythroid (CFU-E) and their offsprings, thereby generating an increased number of normoblasts and, eventually, reticulocytes (Fig. 11.1). Reticulocytosis becomes apparent after a lag of 4 days following an acute increase in the concentration of circulating Epo [8]. Other blood markers of the activation of erythropoiesis are increases in the number of macrocytes and the concentration of soluble transferrin receptor [9].

Hypoxic Induction of Epo Production

On tissue hypoxia, Epo synthesis increases in the kidneys and, to a minor degree, in certain other organs such as the liver and the brain [10]. The expression of the *Epo* gene (chromosome 7q22) is under the control of several transcription factors. GATA-2 inhibits *Epo* expression [11]. Under hypoxic conditions, the binding of GATA-2 to the *Epo* promoter is reduced. Hypoxia-inducible transcription factors (HIF-1 and, most importantly, HIF-2) activate the *Epo* enhancer [12, 13]. The HIFs consist of an O_2-labile α-subunit and a constitutive β-subunit [14]. *Epo* expression is suppressed in normoxia because the HIF-α subunits undergo prolyl and asparaginyl hydroxylation. On prolyl hydroxylation, the von-Hippel–Lindau protein (pVHL) E3

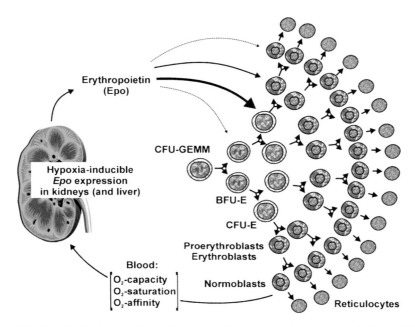

Fig. 11.1 Simplified scheme of the feedback control of erythropoiesis. Lack of O_2 (hypoxia) is a stimulus for the synthesis of erythropoietin (Epo), primarily in the kidneys. Epo is a survival, proliferation, and differentiation factor for the erythrocytic progenitors, particularly the colony-forming units-erythroid (CFU-E). The O_2 capacity of the blood increases with the enhanced release of reticulocytes

ubiquitin ligase complex binds to HIF-α, which is thereupon immediately degraded in the proteasome. Asparaginyl hydroxylation of HIF-α reduces its transcriptional activity by blocking the transcriptional coactivator p300. The HIF-α hydroxylases do not only require O_2 for their catalytic action but also Fe^{2+} and 2-oxoglutarate. Accordingly, the inactivation of HIF-α can be prevented in normoxia by iron depletion or by the application of 2-oxoglutarate competitors (reviewed in ref. [15]).

In persons with intact kidneys and no inflammation, the plasma Epo concentrations increase exponentially with decreasing blood Hb concentrations. Epo values may rise to 10,000 IU/l (International Units per liter) in severe anemia, compared to the normal value of about 15 IU/l. *Epo* expression is also stimulated when the arterial O_2 tension (pO_2) decreases or when the O_2 affinity of the blood is abnormally high. The plasma Epo level increases during acclimatization to high altitude, with peak values 1–2 days after the ascent [16]. Thereafter, erythropoiesis remains to be stimulated although the Epo level is little increased at continued altitude residence [17]. Training and/or residence at altitude (or in artificially O_2-deprived chambers at sea level) have been applied to improve performance in athletes [18–20]. Because exercise under hypoxic conditions impairs training quality [19], the "living high – training low" paradigm has been developed and shown to be effective for athletes of various abilities [19, 20]. Note that the benefit derived from enhanced O_2 capacity is eventually offset by the increase in blood viscosity. Excessive increases in hematocrit (Hct) are of pathogenetic importance in the development of chronic mountain sickness [21].

Effect of Physical Exercise on Erythropoiesis

The plasma Epo level is not generally affected by single bouts of strenuous exercise at sea level as shown following cross-country skiing [22, 23], biathlon [24], cycling [23, 25, 26], and long-distance running [23]. Slight increases were occasionally observed a few hours after long-distance running [27, 28]. The lack of major effects of normoxic exercise on Epo production is plausible, since the O_2 sensor in control of Epo synthesis is not located in skeletal muscle or heart but in the kidneys. Decreases in renal blood flow are unlikely to exert a major influence on *Epo* expression [29]. Plasma Epo levels increase if exercise is performed at altitude [30, 31].

Despite the lack of an increase in circulating Epo during physical exercise at sea level, the number of reticulocytes may increase 1–2 days thereafter [32]. Stress hormones such as catecholamines and cortisol stimulate the release of young red blood cells from the bone marrow. Hb levels and Hct in sportsmen may nevertheless be below normal [33]. This "sports anemia" is truly a pseudoanemia due to an enlarged plasma volume.

Erythropoietic Compounds and Techniques

Epo-R Ligands

The originator rhEpo preparations, Epoetin alfa and Epoetin beta, were engineered in Chinese Hamster Ovary (CHO) cell cultures transfected with the human *Epo* gene, respectively with Epo cDNA. Copies of these products have been produced in many countries outside the US and the EU [34]. Since the patents for the originator Epoetins have expired, biosimilar products ("biosimilars") have been launched in the EU (Table 11.1). To the author's knowledge, the rhEpo (Epoetin omega) engineered in transfected baby hamster kidney (BHK) cell cultures [4] is presently only available in South Africa. The marketing of a humanized rhEpo (Epoetin delta), which was engineered in human fibrosarcoma cells transfected with a viral promoter, has been stopped by the end of 2008. While the amino-acid sequence of all Epoetins is identical with that of endogenous human Epo, their glycosylation pattern varies, as indicated by different Greek letters added to the names [35].

Second-generation ESAs have a long half-life. The mutein Darbepoetin alfa possesses two additional *N*-glycans (in positions 30 and 88), which prolong the terminal half-life on intravenous (i.v.) administration to about 25 h compared to

6–9 h with the Epoetins [36]. Methoxy-PEG-Epo beta, which contains a 30 kDa methoxy-polyethylene glycol polymer at either Ala^1, Lys^{45} or Lys^{52}, has a half-life of about 1 week [37]. rhEpo fusion proteins with additional peptides or the F_c region of human IgG are still in clinical trials (Table 11.1).

Chemically, products in clinical trials include synthetic erythropoiesis protein (SEP) and Epo mimetic peptides (EMPs). EMPs are cyclic peptides of about 20 amino acids which bind to the Epo-R but are unrelated in primary structure to Epo [38]. A pegylated synthetic EMP dimer (Hematide™) increases Hb in healthy persons [39] and may soon be approved for the treatment of anemia in CKD. A novel EMP in clinical trials is CNTO 528, which is attached to human IgG I-based scaffolds by recombinant DNA technology [40].

Table 11.1 Erythropoiesis-stimulating compounds and techniques prohibited in sports

Compound/technique	Manufacturing procedure	Marketing status
Recombinant products		
Originator Epoetin alfa, Epoetin beta	*Epo*-transfected CHO cells	Marketed in EU, North America, Australia, Asia
Epoetin alfa biosimilars ("Epoetin alfa", "Epoetin zeta")	*Epo*-transfected CHO cells	Marketed in EU
Epoetin alfa copies	*Epo*-transfected CHO cells	Marketed in Asia, Central and South America, Africa
Epoetin omega	*Epo*-transfected BHK cells	Marketed in South Africa
Epoetin delta	CMV promoter-transfected HT-1080 cells	No longer available (marketing stopped in 2009)
Methoxy-PEG-Epoetin beta	*Epo*-transfected CHO cells, posttranslational modification	Marketed in EU, Australia and Asia
Darbepoetin alfa	Mutated *Epo*-transfected CHO cells, hyperglycosylated	Marketed in EU, North America, Australia, Asia
Synthetic erythropoiesis protein (SEP)	Chemical synthesis, polymer coupled	In preclinical trials
Epo fusion proteins (Epo-Epo, Epo-Fc, Epo-βHCG)	cDNA-transfected cells	In clinical trials
Epo mimetics		
Peptidic (Hematide™)	Chemical synthesis, PEG coupled	In clinical trials
Nonpeptidic	Chemical synthesis	In preclinical trials
Epo gene activators		
HIF stabilizers	Chemical synthesis	In clinical trials
GATA inhibitors	Chemical synthesis	In preclinical trials
Epo gene transfer		
	In vitro gene transfer	In clinical trials
	In vivo gene transfer	In preclinical trials

Modified from ref. [72]

Stimulators of Endogenous Epo Production

GATA inhibitors are under development that can be taken orally and prevent GATA-2 from suppressing the *Epo* promoter [41]. These nonpeptidic organic compounds increase the acetylation of GATA-2 and enhance the DNA-binding of HIF. GATA inhibitors may be misused in sports, since they were shown to increase Epo concentrations, Hb levels, and endurance performance in mice [42]. Likewise, 2-oxoglutarate analogs (medical jargon "HIF stabilizers") stimulate Epo production in experimental animals [43]. One of these compounds (FG-2216) has been shown to increase plasma Epo levels and reticulocyte numbers in Rhesus macaques [44]. HIF stabilizers induce the expression of >100 genes apart from *Epo*, which may result in serious unwanted effects such as the promotion of tumor growth. Due to the Fe^{2+} requirement of the HIF-α hydroxylases, inactivation of HIF can also be prevented by Fe^{2+} removal. The Fe^{2+} chelator desferrioxamine, which is used therapeutically to reduce chronic iron overload, increases Epo production in man [45, 46]. Cobalt, which displaces Fe^{2+} from the HIF-α hydroxylases, was earlier used to treat anemic CKD patients [47].

Epo Gene Transfer

An autologous ex vivo *Epo* gene therapy trial has already been undertaken on patients with CKD [48]. The reimplantation of dermal core samples transfected with *Epo* cDNA into the skin of the patients resulted in a reticulocytosis but was not sufficient to raise Hb levels [48]. The in vivo *Epo* transfer has not been explored clinically because nonhuman primates develop severe anemia following the viral transfer of *Epo* cDNA due to a break of self-antigen tolerance [49, 50].

Effects of Epo Administration on Physical Performance

The O_2 capacity of the blood can be increased by transfusion of RBC, infusion of Hb, or stimulation of erythropoiesis. RBC transfusion maneuvers increase VO_{2max} and prolong the time to exhaustion on heavy workload [51]. The effects may be partly due to increases in cardiac output and blood buffering capacity. ESAs enhance performance mainly by raising the mass of Hb and RBC while the plasma volume decreases [52, 53]. The subcutaneous (s.c.) administration of rhEpo at total doses of 60–350 IU kg^{-1} body mass $week^{-1}$ for 4–6 weeks increases VO_{2max} and time to exhaustion in exercising male athletes [54–56]. In theory, the rise in Hb mass should be particularly effective during bouts of exercise, such as during sprints and mountain riding in bicycle races. Reportedly, however, the prolonged administration of rhEpo improves submaximal performance more than the aerobic capacity [57].

While Wilkerson et al. [58] found that rhEpo treatment increased VO_{2max} but did not influence VO_2 kinetics on moderate or heavy cycling, Connes et al. [59] observed an acceleration of the dynamic response of VO_2. A study in recreational athletes has shown that following a booster phase (3×50 IU kg^{-1} week^{-1} for 3 weeks), low rhEpo doses (3×20 IU kg^{-1} week^{-1} for another 5 weeks) suffice to maintain Hct and VO_{2max} at 5–10% above the pretreatment levels [60].

Systemically administered rhEpo can cross the blood–brain barrier and exert neuroprotective effects in brain diseases [61]. In male endurance athletes, the treatment with rhEpo (3×50 IU kg^{-1} week^{-1} for 4 weeks followed by 3×20 IU kg^{-1} week^{-1} for 2 weeks) did produce an increase not only in aerobic physical fitness but also in the perceived physical strength scores [62]. This effect can lead to a stronger commitment to training, indicating a potential hedonic desire towards physical burden.

Detection of Doping with ESA

Endogenous Epo (ten isoforms in the isoelectric point (pI) range 3.77–4.70) appearing in urine is generally more acidic [63–65] and smaller in molecular weight [66] than the Epoetins (four to six isoforms in the pI range 4.42–5.21). Darbepoetin alfa migrates more in the acidic range than endogenous human Epo [64, 67]. IEF of urine is commonly performed with 1,000-fold concentrated samples depleted of small molecules by centrifugal ultrafiltration and, possibly, purification on immunoaffinity columns [68]. In the double immunoblotting procedure [3, 67], the proteins in the gel are first transferred to a polyvinylidene fluoride (PVDF) membrane and incubated with anti-Epo monoclonal mouse antibody (mAb; clone AE7A5 [69]). Following the disruption of Epo or Darbepoetin, the mAb is transferred to a second PVDF membrane and incubated with biotinylated secondary antibody for staining with streptavidin-horseradish peroxidase and chemiluminescent substrate [70]. Various biosimilar and copied CHO cell-derived rhEpos are available in the EU, Asia, Central and South America. Because the glycosylation pattern of rhEpo depends on the host cell culture and protein purification procedures [5], the products differ with respect to their behavior on IEF [34, 71]. Methodological weaknesses of the ESA detection method have been discussed elsewhere [72]. In addition, cheating athletes may escape from detection, since only microdoses of rhEpo are needed to maintain elevated Hb levels following a booster phase. In this situation, the window of detection of rhEpo in urine is only 12–18 h [73], compared to about 3 days on regular dosing ($2–3 \times 50$ IU kg^{-1} week^{-1}) [74]. Due to the long half-life of Darbepoetin alfa, the window of detection of this drug is 7 days [75], at least [76]. Due to its high concentrations in blood, Methoxy-PEG-Epo beta is filtered in the renal corpuscles and excreted with the urine in detectable amounts despite the large size of the drug. Methoxy-PEG-Epo beta can be assayed by ELISA including two antibodies, one of which being directed against the Epo molecule and the other to the Methoxy-PEG adduct.

Conclusions

rhEpo and its long-acting analogs and derivatives, which are most beneficial antianemic drugs in clinical practice, have been misused by elite athletes whose desire to win has overcome ethical and medical considerations. The recombinant products can be detected in urine by IEF and immunoblotting, as the structure of their glycan isoforms differs from that of endogenous Epo. However, with several novel erythropoietic drugs entering the market, antidoping control is becoming more difficult. The new compounds include biosimilars of conventional Epoetin alfa, copied products, Epo fusion proteins, and peptidic as well as nonpeptidic Epo mimetics. It is important to establish detection methods prior to the public availability of the drugs. Furthermore, strict out-of-competition testing and long-term storage of urine and blood samples for later investigations are important in the antidoping fight. It is crucial to inform the athletes and their supporting staff of potential health risks of the use of erythropoiesis-stimulating drugs.

To facilitate the detection of blood doping, the WADA has developed recently the "Athlete Biological Passport", which is based on the monitoring of an athlete's biological variables over time, rather than on the traditional direct detection of doping. The Athlete Biological Passport Operating Guidelines were approved by WADA's Executive Committee on December 1, 2009, and took effect immediately.

References

1. Jelkmann W. Erythropoietin: Molecular Biology and Clinical Use. Johnson City: FP Graham Publishing, 2003.
2. Cooper CE. The biochemistry of drugs and doping methods used to enhance aerobic sport performance. Essays Biochem. 2008; 44:63–83.
3. Lasne F. Double-blotting: a solution to the problem of non-specific binding of secondary antibodies in immunoblotting procedures. J Immunol Methods. 2001; 253:125–31.
4. Skibeli V, Nissen-Lie G, Torjesen P. Sugar profiling proves that human serum erythropoietin differs from recombinant human erythropoietin. Blood. 2001; 98:3626–34.
5. Jelkmann W. Recombinant EPO production – points the nephrologist should know. Nephrol Dial Transplant. 2007; 22:2749–53.
6. Yoshimura A, Misawa H. Physiology and function of the erythropoietin receptor. Curr Opin Hematol. 1998; 5:171–6.
7. Richmond TD, Chohan M, Barber DL. Turning cells red: signal transduction mediated by erythropoietin. Trends Cell Biol. 2005; 15:146–55.
8. Major A, Mathez-Loic F, Rohling R, et al. The effect of intravenous iron on the reticulocyte response to recombinant human erythropoietin. Br J Haematol. 1997; 98:292–4.
9. Parisotto R, Gore CJ, Emslie KR, et al. A novel method utilising markers of altered erythropoiesis for the detection of recombinant human erythropoietin abuse in athletes. Haematologica. 2000; 85:564–72.
10. Jelkmann W. Control of erythropoietin gene expression and its use in medicine. Methods Enzymol. 2007; 435:179–97.
11. Imagawa S, Yamamoto M, Miura Y. GATA transcription factors negatively regulate erythropoietin gene expression. Acta Haematol. 1996; 95:248–56.

12. Warnecke C, Zaborowska Z, Kurreck J, et al. Differentiating the functional role of hypoxia-inducible factor (HIF)-1alpha and HIF-2alpha (EPAS-1) by the use of RNA interference: erythropoietin is a HIF-2alpha target gene in Hep3B and Kelly cells. FASEB J. 2004; 18:1462–4.
13. Rankin EB, Biju MP, Liu Q, et al. Hypoxia-inducible factor-2 (HIF-2) regulates hepatic erythropoietin in vivo. J Clin Invest. 2007; 117:1068–77.
14. Wang GL, Jiang BH, Rue EA, et al. Hypoxia-inducible factor 1 is a basic-helix-loop-helix-PAS heterodimer regulated by cellular O_2 tension. Proc Natl Acad Sci USA. 1995; 92:5510–4.
15. Bruegge K, Jelkmann W, Metzen E. Hydroxylation of hypoxia-inducible transcription factors and chemical compounds targeting the HIF-α hydroxylases. Curr Med Chem. 2007; 14:1853–62.
16. Milledge JS, Cotes PM. Serum erythropoietin in humans at high altitude and its relation to plasma renin. J Appl Physiol. 1985; 59:360–4.
17. Monge C, Leon-Velarde F. Physiological adaptation to high altitude: oxygen transport in mammals and birds. Physiol Rev. 1991; 71:1135–72.
18. Favier R, Spielvogel H, Desplanches D, et al. Training in hypoxia vs. training in normoxia in high-altitude natives. J Appl Physiol. 1995; 78:2286–93.
19. Levine BD, Stray-Gundersen J. "Living high-training low": effect of moderate-altitude acclimatization with low-altitude training on performance. J Appl Physiol. 1997; 83:102–12.
20. Stray-Gundersen J, Chapman RF, Levine BD. "Living high-training low" altitude training improves sea level performance in male and female elite runners. J Appl Physiol. 2001; 91:1113–20.
21. Dainiak N, Spielvogel H, Sorba S, et al. Erythropoietin and the polycythemia of high-altitude dwellers. Adv Exp Med Biol. 1989; 271:17–21.
22. Berglund B, Birgegard G, Hemmingsson P. Serum erythropoietin in cross-country skiers. Med Sci Sports Exerc. 1988; 20:208–9.
23. Klausen T, Breum L, Fogh-Andersen N, et al. The effect of short and long duration exercise on serum erythropoietin concentrations. Eur J Appl Physiol Occup Physiol. 1993; 67:213–7.
24. Ricci G, Masotti M, Paoli-Vitali E, et al. Effects of a mixed physical activity (biathlon) on haematologic parameters, red cell 2,3-DPG and creatine, serum erythropoietin, urinary enzymes and microalbumin. Eur J Haematol. 1990; 45:178–9.
25. Schmidt W, Eckardt KU, Hilgendorf A, et al. Effects of maximal and submaximal exercise under normoxic and hypoxic conditions on serum erythropoietin level. Int J Sports Med. 1991; 12:457–61.
26. Gareau R, Caron C, Brisson GR. Exercise duration and serum erythropoietin level. Horm Metab Res. 1991; 23:355.
27. Ricci G, Masotti M, Paoli-Vitali E, et al. Effects of exercise on haematologic parameters, serum iron, serum ferritin, red cell 2,3-diphosphoglycerate and creatine contents, and serum erythropoietin in long-distance runners during basal training. Acta Haematol. 1988; 80:95–8.
28. Schwandt HJ, Heyduck B, Gunga HC, et al. Influence of prolonged physical exercise on the erythropoietin concentration in blood. Eur J Appl Physiol Occup Physiol. 1991; 63:463–6.
29. Pagel H, Jelkmann W, Weiss C. A comparison of the effects of renal artery constriction and anemia on the production of erythropoietin. Pflügers Arch. 1988; 413:62–6.
30. Roberts D, Smith DJ, Donnelly S, et al. Plasma-volume contraction and exercise-induced hypoxaemia modulate erythropoietin production in healthy humans. Clin Sci (Lond). 2000; 98:39–45.
31. Schobersberger W, Hobisch-Hagen P, Fries P, et al. Increase in immune activation, vascular endothelial growth factor and erythropoietin after an ultramarathon run at moderate altitude. Immunobiology. 2000; 201:611–20.
32. Schmidt W, Maassen N, Trost F, et al. Training induced effects on blood volume, erythrocyte turnover and haemoglobin oxygen binding properties. Eur J Appl Physiol Occup Physiol. 1988; 57:490–8.
33. Szygula Z. Erythrocytic system under the influence of physical exercise and training. Sports Med. 1990; 10:181–97.
34. Park SS, Park J, Ko J, et al. Biochemical assessment of erythropoietin products from Asia versus US Epoetin alfa manufactured by Amgen. J Pharm Sci. 2009; 98(5):1688–99.

35. World Health Organization. International nonproprietary names (INN) for biological and biotechnological substances. 2008; http://www.who.int/medicines/services/inn/CompleteBioRevdoc%20 08-11-07_2_pdf.
36. Elliott S, Lorenzini T, Asher S, et al. Enhancement of therapeutic protein in vivo activities through glycoengineering. Nat Biotechnol. 2003; 21:414–21.
37. Macdougall IC. CERA (Continuous Erythropoietin Receptor Activator): a new erythropoiesis-stimulating agent for the treatment of anemia. Curr Hematol Rep. 2005; 4:436–40.
38. Johnson DL, Farrell FX, Barbone FP, et al. Amino-terminal dimerization of an erythropoietin mimetic peptide results in increased erythropoietic activity. Chem Biol. 1997; 4:939–50.
39. Stead RB, Lambert J, Wessels D, et al. Evaluation of the safety and pharmacodynamics of Hematide, a novel erythropoietic agent, in a phase 1, double-blind, placebo-controlled, dose-escalation study in healthy volunteers. Blood. 2006; 108:1830–4.
40. Bouman-Thio E, Franson K, Miller B, et al. A phase I, single and fractionated, ascending-dose study evaluating the safety, pharmacokinetics, pharmacodynamics, and immunogenicity of an erythropoietin mimetic antibody fusion protein (CNTO 528) in healthy male subjects. J Clin Pharmacol. 2008; 48:1197–207.
41. Nakano Y, Imagawa S, Matsumoto K, et al. Oral administration of K-11706 inhibits GATA binding activity, enhances hypoxia-inducible factor 1 binding activity, and restores indicators in an in vivo mouse model of anemia of chronic disease. Blood. 2004; 104:4300–7.
42. Imagawa S, Matsumoto K, Horie M, et al. Does K-11706 enhance performance and why? Int J Sports Med. 2007; 28:928–33.
43. Safran M, Kim WY, O'Connell F, et al. Mouse model for noninvasive imaging of HIF prolyl hydroxylase activity: assessment of an oral agent that stimulates erythropoietin production. Proc Natl Acad Sci USA. 2006; 103(1):105–10.
44. Hsieh MM, Linde NS, Wynter A, et al. HIF prolyl hydroxylase inhibition results in endogenous erythropoietin induction, erythrocytosis, and modest fetal hemoglobin expression in rhesus macaques. Blood. 2007; 110:2140–7.
45. Kling PJ, Dragsten PR, Roberts RA, et al. Iron deprivation increases erythropoietin production in vitro, in normal subjects and patients with malignancy. Br J Haematol. 1996; 95:241–8.
46. Ren X, Dorrington KL, Maxwell PH, et al. Effects of desferrioxamine on serum erythropoietin and ventilatory sensitivity to hypoxia in humans. J Appl Physiol. 2000; 89:680–6.
47. Weissbecker L. Die Kobalttherapie. Dtsch Med Wochenschr. 1950; 75:116–8.
48. Lippin Y, Dranitzki-Elhalel M, Brill-Almon E, et al. Human erythropoietin gene therapy for patients with chronic renal failure. Blood. 2005; 106:2280–6.
49. Gao G, Lebherz C, Weiner DJ, et al. Erythropoietin gene therapy leads to autoimmune anemia in macaques. Blood. 2004; 103:3300–2.
50. Chenuaud P, Larcher T, Rabinowitz JE, et al. Autoimmune anemia in macaques following erythropoietin gene therapy. Blood. 2004; 103:3303–4.
51. Gaudard A, Varlet-Marie E, Bressolle F, et al. Drugs for increasing oxygen and their potential use in doping: a review. Sports Med. 2003; 33:187–212.
52. Lundby C, Thomsen JJ, Boushel R, et al. Erythropoietin treatment elevates haemoglobin concentration by increasing red cell volume and depressing plasma volume. J Physiol. 2007; 578:309–14.
53. Lundby C, Robach P, Boushel R, et al. Does recombinant human Epo increase exercise capacity by means other than augmenting oxygen transport? J Appl Physiol. 2008; 105:581–7.
54. Ekblom B, Berglund B. Effect of erythropoietin administration on maximal aerobic power in man. Scand J Med Sci Sports. 1991; 1:88–93.
55. Audran M, Gareau R, Matecki S, et al. Effects of erythropoietin administration in training athletes and possible indirect detection in doping control. Med Sci Sports Exerc. 1999; 31:639–45.
56. Birkeland KI, Stray-Gundersen J, Hemmersbach P, et al. Effect of rhEPO administration on serum levels of sTfR and cycling performance. Med Sci Sports Exerc. 2000; 32:1238–43.
57. Thomsen JJ, Rentsch RL, Robach P, et al. Prolonged administration of recombinant human erythropoietin increases submaximal performance more than maximal aerobic capacity. Eur J Appl Physiol. 2007; 101:481–6.

58. Wilkerson DP, Rittweger J, Berger NJ, et al. Influence of recombinant human erythropoietin treatment on pulmonary O_2 uptake kinetics during exercise in humans. J Physiol. 2005; 568:639–52.
59. Connes P, Perrey S, Varray A, et al. Faster oxygen uptake kinetics at the onset of submaximal cycling exercise following 4 weeks recombinant human erythropoietin (r-HuEPO) treatment. Pflügers Arch. 2003; 447:231–8.
60. Russell G, Gore CJ, Ashenden MJ, et al. Effects of prolonged low doses of recombinant human erythropoietin during submaximal and maximal exercise. Eur J Appl Physiol. 2002; 86:442–9.
61. Siren AL, Fasshauer T, Bartels C, et al. Therapeutic potential of erythropoietin and its structural or functional variants in the nervous system. Neurotherapeutics. 2009; 6:108–27.
62. Ninot G, Connes P, Caillaud C. Effects of recombinant human erythropoietin injections on physical self in endurance athletes. J Sports Sci. 2006; 24:383–91.
63. Lasne F, de Ceaurriz J. Recombinant erythropoietin in urine. Nature. 2000; 405:635.
64. Catlin DH, Breidbach A, Elliott S, et al. Comparison of the isoelectric focusing patterns of darbepoetin alfa, recombinant human erythropoietin, and endogenous erythropoietin from human urine. Clin Chem. 2002; 48:2057–9.
65. Pascual JA, Belalcazar V, de Bolos C, et al. Recombinant erythropoietin and analogues: a challenge for doping control. Ther Drug Monit. 2004; 26:175–9.
66. Kohler M, Ayotte C, Desharnais P, et al. Discrimination of recombinant and endogenous urinary erythropoietin by calculating relative mobility values from SDS gels. Int J Sports Med. 2008; 29:1–6.
67. Lasne F, Martin L, Crepin N, et al. Detection of isoelectric profiles of erythropoietin in urine: differentiation of natural and administered recombinant hormones. Anal Biochem. 2002; 311:119–26.
68. Lasne F, Martin L, Martin J, et al. Isoelectric profiles of human erythropoietin are different in serum and urine. Int J Biol Macromol. 2007; 41:354–7.
69. Sytkowski AJ, Fisher JW. Isolation and characterization of an anti-peptide monoclonal antibody to human erythropoietin. J Biol Chem. 1985; 260:14727–31.
70. WADA. Harmonization of the method for the identification of Epoetin alfa and beta (EPO) and Darbepoetin alfa (NESP) by IEF-double blotting and chemiluminescent detection. 2007; www.wada-ama.org/rtecontent/document/td2007epo_en.pdf.
71. Schellekens H. Biosimilar epoetins: how similar are they? Eur J Hosp Pharm. 2004; 3:43–47.
72. Jelkmann W. Erythropoiesis stimulating agents and techniques: a challenge for doping analysts. Curr Med Chem. 2009; 16(10):1236–47.
73. Ashenden M, Varlet-Marie E, Lasne F, et al. The effects of microdose recombinant human erythropoietin regimens in athletes. Haematologica. 2006; 91:1143–4.
74. Breidbach A, Catlin DH, Green GA, et al. Detection of recombinant human erythropoietin in urine by isoelectric focusing. Clin Chem. 2003; 49:901–7.
75. Lamon S, Robinson N, Mangin P, et al. Detection window of Darbepoetin-alpha following one single subcutaneous injection. Clin Chim Acta. 2007; 379:145–9.
76. Morkeberg J, Lundby C, Nissen-Lie G, et al. Detection of darbepoetin alfa misuse in urine and blood: a preliminary investigation. Med Sci Sports Exerc. 2007; 39:1742–7.

Chapter 12
Amino Acids and Nonhormonal Compounds for Doping in Athletes

Zvi Zadik

Nutritional abuse may be defined as large doses of supplements in athletes above those taken for nutritional purposes. This definition is vague especially since there is still disagreement on the right required physiologic needs of athletes.

Many athletes start their career at an age when growth and maturity are not completed yet. Physiologic and metabolic needs at this age are different from those of adults [1].

It is Difficult to Draw the Line Between Special Needs and Doping

In adults, since the rapid growth period is over, and de novo synthesis of new tissue is no longer an accelerated process, it has been suggested that a well-balanced isocaloric diet is sufficient to guarantee basic macro- and micronutrients requirements for the majority of athletes [2–4]. This general agreement has acceptations. However, some athletes may need "supplements" that replace essential nutrients missing from their regular diet. Special needs like fluids and salt during special climatic circumstances (humidity, temperature, etc.) [5] and increased need for calories or protein intake without fat causes us to choose concentrated amino acids [3]. Certain sports, taking into consideration the sport's type, intensity, and frequency, may need a change in nutritional supplementation. On these occasions, of special needs, these supplements cannot be considered as nutritional abuse, provided the supplement is given so that it reaches the physiological needed doses of the nutrient.

Z. Zadik (✉)
Chairman Research Authority, Kaplan Medical Center, Rehovot, Israel
and
School of Nutritional Sciences, Hebrew University, Rehovot, Israel
e-mail: zvizadik@012.net.il

E. Ghigo et al. (eds.), *Hormone Use and Abuse by Athletes*, Endocrine Updates 29,
DOI 10.1007/978-1-4419-7014-5_12, © Springer Science+Business Media, LLC 2011

In addition to a proper training program, adequate nutrition can make the difference between success and failure. The main problem is that most of the "theories" on food supplements are not evidence based. For example, while for certain substances physiologic effects were demonstrated by parenteral route, the main use of these substances is as an oral food additive. When demonstrating a theoretical physiological role of a substance, we still have to demonstrate its long-acting effect and more importantly its efficiency to sport. As in the case of amino acids, the administration of arginine and other amino acids stimulate growth hormone secretion [6] via inhibition of GH response to growth-hormone-releasing hormone by somatostatin secretion [7]. This is the logic behind amino-acid supplement. Yet, the oral doses of arginine taken for this purpose are so much higher than the parenteral dose, so that they cause gastrointestinal problems. Despite the theoretical logic of amino-acid administration, no effect on muscle function was demonstrated. The same stands for other substances taken in mega doses like vitamins and minerals. A more complicated issue is the "natural products" sold in different forms as extracts, powders, herbs, etc. with no good quality control on their ingredients and contaminants (as hormones).

Lack of evidence on the real effectiveness and usefulness of "ergogenic" supplements are the result of two main reasons: (1) Controlled research might damage the huge market of the substances that are sold anyway (2) The production of ergogenic substances for improving sport achievements is illegal. The result is that we are left with a population of athletes taking mega doses of nutrients commonly found in the normal human diet or "enhancers" without much knowledge on possible health risks and without knowledge on the maximal daily total safe dose of all these substances. Since these are normal ingredients of our daily diet, there is no efficient way to control intake or to relate to them as prohibited substances.

As reported in literature, supplements are currently used in an attempt to increase sport performance in various ways, such as providing an increased energy supply, increased energy-releasing muscular metabolic processes, enhanced oxygen delivery to active muscles, increased oxygen use, decreased accumulation of fatigue-related substances, and improved neural control of muscle contraction [8].

It is to remember that even natural products and food supplements that are "clean" and not contaminated with hormones might have secondary effects on hormonal systems as photochemical, phytoestrogens, plants sterols, different herbs, etc.

Different surveys on the use of supplements report that 40–60% of athletes take food additives, and the number is rapidly increasing. About 50% of the recommendations to use these supplements come from nonprofessional people.

Proteins as Supplements

Proteins are one of the most popular additives given to athletes and body builders.

Disputes on the proper required supplement still exist as summarized by Philips [9]. Studies in which protein requirements have been examined in athletes have shown an increased requirement for protein in strength- and endurance-trained athletes.

The increase in requirement has to cover the need to synthesize new muscle or repair muscle damage and to replace marked increase in usage of certain amino acids like leucine that are oxidized. It is important to note that high-protein diets have been shown to be effective in promoting weight reduction, particularly fat loss and preservation of lean mass as compared with lower protein diets. Excessive protein overload may prevent weight gain and growth in certain children and adolescents. A combination of high-protein overload and insufficient calories may cause irreversible damage to growth. On the other hand, it is suggested that the protein requirements of adolescent athletes are above the RDA for nonactive male adolescents [10]. The growing adolescent has different needs. A balance between the sport needs and growth and developmental needs has to be set as presented recently by Nemet and Eliakim [11]. Amino acids are frequently used since they are easier to absorb than proteins.

Amino acids as Supplements

Amino acids (AA) have an effect on different control mechanisms of hormone secretion and metabolic pathways. A part of the AA ingested might be used as a source of energy.

Branched chain AA supplementation stimulates basal insulin synthesis and secretion and increases insulin-sensitivity, without modifying the insulin response to acute physical exercise [12].

While overloading a single amino acid in a clinical trial, we never get a net effect of that amino acid, as transport mechanisms are common for few amino acids. So, an overload of one amino acid inhibits the transport of others and at the same time may inhibit the effect of other AA. In addition, an amino acid may have a widespread effect on the brain and endocrine system at different levels and by various mechanisms as control of the pituitary gland through neurotransmitter systems influencing pituitary hormone secretion and changing the metabolic control of CNS. Changes in neurotransmitter systems may cause behavioral changes. Certain amino acids exert a specific excitatory activity at brain level [13]. Different reports on the use of a single amino acid and combination experiments make us speculate that dietary AA might influence basal and stress related hormonal levels. The whole picture is not clear yet.

AA Involvement in the Control of Neurotransmitter System

AA might have an effect on the control mechanisms of the endocrine system as pituitary secretion. The availability of the AA tyrosine, phenylalanine, and tryptophan influence the rate of synthesis of catecholaminergic and serotonergic system neurotransmitters. The availability of these AA depends on a transport mechanism that is affected by isoleucine, leucine, methionine, and valine which use the same transport systems and therefore may have an effect on the rate of uptake of their amino acid precursors from the circulation. These AA have to cross the blood–brain barrier via a membrane-bound transport system (large neutral amino-acid transporter). The uptake of these AA is affected by the plasma levels of other AA competing for uptake into the brain via the same transport mechanism. This mechanism is critical for understanding that the result of an AA overload might be inhibition or change of a known effect of another AA. These mechanisms are involved not only in pituitary hormone secretion but also in behavioral changes important to athletes. For example, branched chain AA was reported as responsible for reducing fatigue in athletes [14].

Effects on Pituitary Hormones GH, ACTH, LH, FSH and on Sex Steroids [15–18]

Examples for the effects of single amino acid on hormone secretion: glutamic acid on ACTH and cortisol, ornhitine on ACTH, cortisol, and GH. Branched chain AA were reported to increase testosterone and cortisol in a single administration during physical exercise. Long-term use of branched chain AA induced increases in plasma cortisol and testosterone.

As presented earlier, AA might influence the pituitary secretion directly at the hypothalamic–pituitary level, or through modification of the neuroendocrine system that regulates hormonal and metabolic pathways, such as catecholamines for example. An additional indirect influential way is AA production of substances that influence hormonal secretion or activity, as in the case of nitric oxide production from arginine by nitric oxide synthetase. Nitric oxide takes part in the regulation of gonadotrophic axis, pituitary adrenal axis, and more.

Indirect Metabolic Effects of AA

In studies of L-glutamate uptake into nonsynaptic mitochondria, isolated from rat cerebral hemispheres, it was demonstrated that arginine functions as a specific modulator of cerebral mitochondrial glutamate transport [19].

The complexity of actions and the diversity of effects on a variety of hormones and mechanisms make it difficult to evaluate the action of a single AA.

Many of the actions were demonstrated in laboratory animals, but not in humans. Some of these actions were tested by parenteral use, but the products sold are for an unproven oral use.

A far reaching practical use not proven yet is the use of arginine (arginine alpha-glutarate) for nitric oxide production. Theoretically, it may improve work capacity, increase muscle growth, and decrease muscle recovery time. No studies have been performed yet to prove these points, nor on improved performance.

Adverse Effects of AA

Safety margins for AA supplements are not yet set. Serious adverse events were reported for L-tryptophan and phenyl alanine. A systemic connective tissue-like disease with close to 50 death cases was reported. The disease was reported as eosinophylia–myalgia syndrome.

Vitamins

Vitamins vary widely in their potential for adverse effects. The difference between a safe low dose and a toxic higher dose is quite large for some vitamins and quite small for others. When used consistently with the Recommended Dietary Allowances (RDA), they are generally considered safe for the general population.

Vitamin A

High doses (>25,000 IU) and in some populations (children, people with liver disease) are associated with severe liver injury-cirrhosis, bone and cartilage pathologies, and pseudotumor cerebri (increased intracranial pressure). Milder forms of disease were reported even on lower doses that were above the RDA.

Vitamin B_6 (Pyridoxine)

High doses above the RDA may cause neurotoxicity, including ataxia and sensory neuropathy.

Niacin (Nicotinic Acid and Nicotinamide)

High doses have been associated with gastrointestinal distress (burning pain, nausea, vomiting, bloating, cramping, and diarrhea) and mild to severe liver damage. In some cases, liver injury, myopathy, eye maculopathy, blood pancytopenia and coagulopathy, hypotensive myocardial infarction, and metabolic acidosis were reports.

Carnitine

Carnitine supplementation is the focus of research for about 25 years. Since it is known that skeletal muscle carnitine deficiency is associated with profound impairment of muscle function, it has been logical to presume that carnitine supplementation can improve skeletal muscle function and athletic performance in healthy individuals. Carnitine, a derivative of beta-hydroxybutyrate, is synthesized mainly in the liver and kidneys from the two essential amino acids, lysine and methionine. Vitamin B_6, nicotinic acids, vitamin C, and folate are also essential for its production. Other tissues that require carnitine, such as muscle, are dependent on transport systems that mediate its export from the liver and uptake by other tissues.

Carnitine has an importance for β-oxidation of fatty acids by facilitating the transport of long-chain fatty acids across the mitochondrial membrane as acylcarnitine esters. Carnitine is also important for glucose metabolism. In carnitine deficiency, fat oxidation and energy production from fatty acids are markedly impaired, and some degree of hypoglycemia might be present.

Trying to summarize data on how much evidence on the usefulness of carnitine as a supplement [20], it appears that there is not enough information on how much carnitine is required to support optimal metabolism in skeletal muscle, how efficiently can oral carnitine supplement increase skeletal muscle carnitine, and how much can carnitine supplementation alter energy homeostasis in healthy subjects, and the last but not the least that there is no convincing evidence that carnitine supplementation can improve physical performance in healthy, nutritionally sufficient athletes. In two recent placebo-controlled trials, Broad et al found no effect on fat, carbohydrate, and protein contribution to metabolism during prolonged moderate-intensity cycling exercise. A tendency toward suppressed ammonia made them to raise the possibility that oral L-carnitine L-tartrate supplementation might have the potential to reduce the metabolic stress of exercise or alter ammonia production or removal [21]. Smith et al. reported that 8 weeks of 3 g/day glycine propionyl-L-carnitine supplementation had no effective increase in muscle carnitine content and no significant effects on aerobic- or anaerobic-exercise performance [22].

Antioxidants

During strenuous exercise, aerobic and anaerobic, oxygen consumption increases, and free-radical production is increased [23]. Exercise mode, intensity, and duration, as well as the population tested, and the nutrition they are on, all may have an impact on the extent of free radical production, since different types of athletic activity differ in their energy use, oxygen consumption, and free-radical production [24]. Muscle damage occurs as a result of the combination of several mechanisms as increased lipid peroxidation, stress-induced catecholamine production, lactic acid production, and inflammatory responses. The damage may occur when free-radical load exceeds the antioxidant potential of the tissue involved [25]. This process may have also an impact on exercise performance through a combination of impairment of muscle contractility and muscle damage [26, 27]. The antioxidant defense system depends on endogenous antioxidant compounds such as glutathione and dietary intake of antioxidant vitamins C and E, beta-carotene, and minerals which are abundant mostly in vegetarian diet [28–40].

Vitamin E is the major antioxidant in cell membranes. It protects against lipid peroxidation by acting directly with a variety of oxygen radicals [41]. Vitamin C can interact with the tocopherol radical to regenerate reduced tocopherol and react with superoxide, hydroxyl radicals, and singlet oxygen. Singlet oxygen is an energized but uncharged form of oxygen that is produced during a "metabolic burst" with a toxic effect on cells [42]. Beta-carotene, the major carotenoid precursor of vitamin A, is the most efficient agent against singlet oxygen [43]. An additional protection mechanism is glutathione peroxidase, an enzyme that functions to remove hydrogen peroxide. Glutathione peroxidase and other antioxidant enzymes (e.g., superoxide dismutases, catalase, and glutathione reductase) function to reduce lipid peroxidation. It is thought that during exercise changes in blood amounts and changes in glutathione antioxidants like vitamins C and E and others are mobilized from tissue stores into the blood to combat oxidative stress. In recent years, studies have reported conflicting results following antioxidant supplementation as summarized recently in an extensive review [44]. While oxidative stress and free-radical production have the potential to result in tissue damage, not all experiments on antioxidant supplementation proved to be beneficial. These conflicting results raised the theoretical possibility that oxidative stress may actually serve as stimulus for the upregulation of antioxidant defenses and recovery against tissue damage. As for physical performance, studies have generally found no beneficial effect of antioxidant therapy. It appears that since trained athletes show less evidence of damage than do untrained subjects, physical training may maximize training-induced adaptations and enhance the antioxidant defense system in addition to physical performance.

Beta-Hydroxy Beta-Methylbutyrate

Strenuous physical activity leads to muscle damage as evidenced by both clinical as muscle soreness [45] and biochemical markers as creatine kinase [45, 46], lactate dehydrogenase (LDH) [47], 3-methylhistidine (3-MH) [46], urine urea nitrogen, and plasma urea [48]. The administration of beta-hydroxy beta-methylbutyrate (HMB) leads to a significant decrease in these markers. It was demonstrated that HMB exerts its effect through increased conversion to 3-hydroxy-3-methylglutaryl-coenzyme A and as a result repair of the sarcolemma following muscle damage that occurs during strenuous exercise [46, 49]. HMB effectiveness was demonstrated during different physical activity protocols [45, 46, 48, 50–52]. Most of the studies have administered HMB for at least 2 weeks prior to strenuous physical activity. Probably, HMB "muscle loading" for the purpose of muscle "saturation" is time- and dose-dependent [46, 53]. Agreement about the most efficient protocol for this purpose was not reached yet.

References

1. Almquist J, Valovich McLeod TC, Cavanna A, Jenkinson D, Lincoln AE, Loud K, et al. Summary statement: appropriate medical care for the secondary school-aged athlete. J Athl Train. 2008;43:416–427.
2. Maughan RJ. Nutritional ergogenic aids and exercise performance. Nutr Res Rev. 1999;12:255–280.
3. Maughan RJ, King DS, Trevor L. Dietary supplements. J Sports Sci. 2004;22:95–113.
4. Volpe SL. Micronutrient requirements for athletes. Clin Sports Med. 2007;26:119–130.
5. Striegel H, Simon P, Wurster C, et al. The use of nutritional supplements among master athletes. Int J Sports Med. 2006;27:236–241.
6. Isidori A, Lo Monaco A, Cappa M. A study of growth hormone release in men after administration of amino acids. Curr Med Res Opin. 1981;7:475–481.
7. Alba RJ, Albrecht Muller O. Arginine stimulates growth hormone secretion by suppressing endogenous somatostatin secretion. J Clin Endocrinol Metab. 1988;67:1186–1189.
8. Williams MH, Leutholtz BC. Nutritional ergogenic aids. In: Maughan R, ed. Nutrition in sport. Oxford: Blackwell Science; 2000:356–366.
9. Phillips SM. Dietary protein for athletes: from requirements to metabolic advantage. Appl Physiol Nutr Metab. 2006;31:647–654.
10. Boisseau N, Vermorel M, Rance M, Duché P, Patureau-Mirand P. Protein requirements in male adolescent soccer players. Eur J Appl Physiol. 2007;100:27–33.
11. Nemet D, Eliakim A. Pediatric sport nutrition – an update. Curr Opin Clin Nutr Metab Care. 2009;12:304–309.
12. Carli G, Bonifazi M, Lodi L. Changes in the exercise induced hormone response to branched chain amino acids administration. Eur J Appl Physiol. 1992;64:272–277.
13. Hicks TP, Conti F. Amino acids as the source of considerable excitation in cerebral cortex. Can J Physiol Pharmacol. 1996;74:341–361.
14. Blomstrand E, Celsing F, Newsholme EA. Changes in plasma concentrations of aromatic and branched-chain amino acid during sustained exercise in men and their possible role in fatigue. Acta Physiol Scand. 1988;133:115–121.
15. Carli G, Bonifazi M, Lodi L, et al. Changes in the exercise induced hormone response to branched chain amino acids administration. Eur J Appl Physiol. 1992;64:272–277.
16. Di Luigi L, Pigozzi F, Casini A, et al. Effects of prolonged amino acid supplementations on hormonal secretion in male athletes. Med Sport. 1994;47:529–539.
17. Evain-Brion D, Donnadieu M, Roger M, et al. Simultaneous study of somatotrophic and corticotrophic pituitary secretion during ornithine infusion test. Clin Endocrinol. 1982;17:119–122.
18. Tegelman R, Johansson C, Hemmingsson P, Eklöf R, Carlström K, Pousette A. Endogenous anabolic and catabolic steroids hormones in male and female athletes during off season. Int J Sports Med. 1990;11:103–106.
19. Dolinska M, Albrecht J. Glutamate uptake is inhibited by L-arginine in mitochondria isolated from rat cerebrum. Neuroreport. 1997;8:2365–2368.
20. Brass EP. Carnitine and sports medicine: use or abuse? Ann N Y Acad Sci. 2004;1033: 67–78.
21. Broad EM, Maughan RJ, Galloway SD. Carbohydrate, protein, and fat metabolism during exercise after oral carnitine supplementation in humans. J Sport Nutr Exerc Metab. 2008;18: 567–584.
22. Smith WA, Fry AC, Tschume LC, Bloomer RJ. Effect of glycine propionyl-L-carnitine on aerobic and anaerobic exercise performance. Int J Sport Nutr Exerc Metab. 2008;18:19–36.
23. Dillard CJ, Litov RE, Savin WM, Dumelin EE, Tappel AL. Effects of exercise, vitamin E, and ozone on pulmonary function and lipid peroxidation. J Appl Physiol. 1978;45(6):927–932.
24. Jackson MJ. Exercise and oxygen radical production by muscle. In: Sen CK, Packer L, Hanninen O, eds. Handbook of oxidants and antioxidants in exercise. Amsterdam: Elsevier Science 2000:57–68.

25. Halliwell B. Oxygen radicals: a commonsense look at their nature and medical importance. Med Biol. 1984;62(2):71–77.
26. Reid MB. Nitric oxide, reactive oxygen species, and skeletal muscle contraction. Med Sci Sports Exerc. 2001;33(3):371–376.
27. Goldhaber JI, Qayyum MS. Oxygen free radicals and excitation–contraction coupling. Antioxid Redox Signal. 2000;2(1):55–64.
28. Halliwell B, Cross CE. Oxygen-derived species: their relation to human disease and environmental stress. Environ Health Perspect 1994;102(Suppl 10):5–12.
29. Aruoma OI. Free radicals and antioxidant strategies in sport. J Nutr Biochem. 1994;5: 370–381.
30. Ji LL. Oxidative stress during exercise: implication of antioxidant nutrients. Free Radic Biol Med. 1995;18:1079–1086.
31. Tiidus PM, Houston ME. Vitamin E status and response to exercise training. Sports Med. 1995;20:12–23.
32. Clarkson PM. Antioxidants and physical performance. Clin Rev Food Sci Nutr. 1995;35: 131–141.
33. Maxwell SRJ. Prospects for the use of antioxidant therapies. Drugs. 1995;49:345–361.
34. Sen CK. Oxidants and antioxidants in exercise. J Appl Physiol. 1995;675:79–86.
35. Dekkers JC, van Doornen LJP, Kemper HCG. The role of antioxidant vitamins and enzymes in the prevention of exercise-induced muscle damage. Sports Med. 1996;21:213–238.
36. Packer L. Oxidants, antioxidant nutrients and the athlete. J Sports Sci. 1997;15:353–363.
37. Ashton T, Rowlands CC, Jones E, et al. Electron spin resonance spectroscopic detection of oxygen-centered radicals in human serum following exhaustive exercise. Eur J Appl Physiol. 1998;77:498–502.
38. Kanter M. Free radicals, exercise and antioxidant supplementation. Proc Nutr Soc. 1998;57:9–13.
39. Urso ML, Clarkson PM. Oxidative stress, exercise, and antioxidant supplementation. Toxicology. 2003;189(1–2):41–54.
40. Watson TA, Callister R, Taylor RD, Sibbritt DW, MacDonald-Wicks LK, Garg ML. Antioxidant restriction and oxidative stress in short-duration exhaustive exercise. Med Sci Sports Exerc. 2005;37(1):63–71.
41. Knez WL, Coombes JS, Jenkins DG. Ultra-endurance exercise and oxidative damage: implications for cardiovascular health. Sports Med. 2006;36(5):429–441.
42. Sauberlich HE. Ascorbic acid. In: Brown ML, ed. Present knowledge in nutrition. Washington, DC: International Life Sciences Institute; 1990:132–141.
43. Olson JA, Vitamin A. In: Brown ML, ed. Present knowledge in nutrition. Washington, DC: International Life Sciences Institute; 1990:96–107.
44. Fisher-Wellman K, Bloomer RJ. Acute exercise and oxidative stress: a 30 year history. Dynamic Medicine. 2009;8:1–25.
45. van Someren KA, Edwards AJ, Howatson G. Supplementation with beta-hydroxy-beta-methylbutyrate (HMB) and alpha-ketoisocaproic acid (KIC) reduces signs and symptoms of exercise-induced muscle damage in man. Int J Sport Nutr Exerc Metab. 2005;15(4):413–424.
46. Nissen S, Sharp R, Ray M, Rathmacher JA, Rice D, Fuller JC Jr. Effect of leucine metabolite beta-hydroxy-beta-methylbutyrate on muscle metabolism during resistance-exercise training. J Appl Physiol. 1996;81:2095–2104.
47. Nitter AE, Panton L, Rathmacher JA, Petersen A, Sharp R. Effects of beta-hydroxy-beta-methylbutyrate on muscle damage after a prolonged run. J Appl Physiol. 2000;89(4): 1340–1344.
48. Jowko E, Ostaszewski P, Jank M, Sacharuk J, Zieniewicz A, Wilczak J. Creatine and beta-hydroxy-beta-methylbutyrate (HMB) additively increase lean body mass and muscle strength during a weight-training program. Nutrition. 2001;17:558–566.
49. Wilson GJ, Wilson JM, Manninen AH. Effects of beta-hydroxy-beta-methylbutyrate (HMB) on exercise performance and body composition across varying levels of age, sex, and training experience: a review. Nutr Metab. 2008;5:1.

50. Gallagher PM, Carrithers JA, Godard MP, Schulze KE, Trappe SW. Beta-hydroxy-beta-methylbutyrate ingestion, part I: effects on strength and fat free mass. Med Sci Sports Exerc. 2000;32:2109–2115.
51. Vukovich MD, Stubbs NB, Bohlken RM. Body composition in 70-year-old adults responds to dietary beta-hydroxy-beta-methylbutyrate similarly to that of young adults. J Nutr. 2001;131: 2049–2052.
52. Panton LB, Rathmacher JA, Baier S, Nissen S. Nutritional supplementation of the leucine metabolite beta-hydroxy-beta-methylbutyrate (hmb) during resistance training. Nutrition. 2000;16:734–739.
53. Neighbors KL, Ransone JW, Jacobson BH, LeFavi RG. Effects of dietary β-hydroxy-β-methylbutyrate on body composition in collegiate football players. Med Sci Sports Exerc. 2000;32:S60.

Chapter 13
The Assay of Endogenous and Exogenous Anabolic Androgenic Steroids

Maria Kristina Parr, Ulrich Flenker, and Wilhelm Schänzer

Introduction

According to the regulations of the World Anti-Doping Agency (WADA) [1], anabolic androgenic steroids are classified as prohibited substances in sports. They are covered in the section "S1. Anabolic Agents 1. Anabolic Androgenic Steroids (AAS)". This section is further subdivided into "a. Exogenous AAS" and "b. Endogenous AAS". AAS represent the class of substances most frequently detected in human sports doping control analyses for many years [2]. The analysis for AAS in doping control is generally performed using urine specimen as matrix.

Most of the AAS are extensively metabolized in the human body and only small amounts of the parent substances are excreted in the urine. The most important metabolic phase-I reactions include oxidation or reduction in positions C-3 and C-17. Furthermore, Δ4 steroids in general are substrates for 5α reduction. Additional double bonds in ring A or B or additional substituents in position C-4 or C-6 push the reduction toward 5β orientation. The introduction of hydroxy functions and their subsequent oxidation especially in positions C-4, C-6, and C-16 is also observed and found most abundantly in steroids like metandienone, dehydrochloromethyltestosterone, stanozolol, and other steroids with additional condensed heterocycles on the A-ring [3–10]. Phase-II metabolism of AAS in humans includes mainly 3α-glucuronidation, while sulfatation mainly occurs at 3β-hydroxy functions. On 17-hydroxy functions, sulfatation as well as glucuronidation occurs equally.

In case of 17-alkylated steroids, 17-epimerization occurs by hydrolysis of the phase-II metabolite, 17-sulfate. As a by-product of this reaction, 17,17-dimethyl-18-nor-13-ene analogs are also detectable [11].

Endogenous AAS represent a special group of compounds. In a strict sense, the relevant steroids are not truly endogenous but are obtained by partial synthesis from plant sterols [12]. The number of compounds with potential of abuse is comparably restricted. Testosterone, biologically the most important anabolic androgenic hormone, is still

M.K. Parr (✉)
Institute of Biochemistry, German Sport University Cologne, Cologne, Germany
e-mail: m.parr@biochem.dshs-koeln.de

E. Ghigo et al. (eds.), *Hormone Use and Abuse by Athletes*, Endocrine Updates 29, DOI 10.1007/978-1-4419-7014-5_13, © Springer Science+Business Media, LLC 2011

likely to be the molecule with the highest potential of abuse. Dehydroepiandrosterone (DHEA), androst-4-ene-3,17-dione, and androst-5-ene-3,17-dione constitute so-called pro-hormones which after application are metabolized to testosterone. On principle, this mimics the physiological situation and the conversion generally follows the biological pathway. As with xenobiotic steroids, mostly oxidations or reductions at positions 3 and 17 occur where the direction is controlled by substrate concentration. Consequently, also androstenediols may serve as pro-hormones.

Finally, the reactions mentioned above result in the formation of testosterone where the physiological yields may differ. In case of the application of $\Delta 5$ compounds, these are converted to the corresponding $\Delta 4$ isomers beforehand.

Boldenone, nortestosterone, and their pro-hormones could be classified as either endogenous or exogenous AAS. They may be synthesized physiologically in very small concentrations. Most likely, these steroids are by-products of the steroid metabolism. In spite of their anabolic and androgenic effects, they can hardly be said to truly represent natural hormones.

Phase-I and phase-II metabolism generally proceed as described above. The reduction of the double bond at position 4 is the initial and also rate-limiting step [13]. This step often is accompanied by the loss of biological activity. The most abundant metabolites following application of testosterone or testosterone pro-hormones are 3α-hydroxy-5α-androstan-17-one (androsterone), 3α-hydroxy-5β-androstan-17-one (etiocholanolone), and the corresponding 17β-diols.

Evidently, classical chemical methodology is incapable of discriminating synthetic hormones from the biosynthesized congeners. However, stable isotope analysis at the natural abundance level represents a powerful way to meet this goal [14–19]. There seem to exist very few sources of raw sterols that serve as educts for partial synthesis of pharmaceutical steroid preparations [12]. Mostly, yams (*Dioscorea* sp.) and soy (*Glycine max*) are used. Both plants feature what is known as the C-3 photosynthetic pathway [20, 21]. This results in a relatively strong depletion of ^{13}C versus atmospheric CO_2. By contrast, humans typically feed on a large variety of foodstuff including seafood and so-called C-4 plants, such as corn (*Zea mays*) and sorghum (*Sorghum* sp.). The $^{13}C/^{12}C$ ratio of this dietary mixture is slightly but significantly larger than that of purely C-3 plant-borne steroids. Based on these distinct isotope signatures, a discrimination of synthetic and natural hormones can be achieved. The signature also propagates into urinary metabolites of steroid hormones. This is advantageous as, for example, testosterone itself is typically found in urine in only small concentrations.

In order to compensate for baseline variations and uncertainties of the calibration, the $^{13}C/^{12}C$ ratios of AAS and corresponding metabolites are not evaluated directly. Instead, the $^{13}C/^{12}C$ ratios of target compounds are compared to those of steroids from androgen-independent pathways.

Sample Preparation

The methods routinely used in steroid screening mainly focus on those metabolites that are excreted in the unconjugated form or as glucuronides with the urine. Common procedures include deconjugation using the β-glucuronidase enzyme derived from *Escherichia coli*. Less frequently, β-glucuronidase/arylsulfatase from *Helix pomatia* is used. Extraction of the aglycons from the matrix and concentration of the analytes is performed by liquid–liquid extraction or solid-phase extraction. To cover the significant diversity of steroids by a single method and to provide high specificity and sensitivity, mass spectrometric methods are utilized for the detection. The final residues are either redissolved in buffer solutions for LC–MS(/MS) analysis or silylated for GC–MS(/MS) analyses. As proposed by Donike et al. [22], most of the laboratories use *N*-methyl-*N*-trimethylsilyl-trifluoroacetamide (MSTFA) as reagent for derivatization. The formation of per-TMS derivatives utilizing trimethyliodosilane as catalyst has proven to drastically improve the sensitivity for most of the steroids in gas chromatography–mass spectrometry (GC–MS) based assays [23, 24]. Several compounds, most of them deuterated, composing the internal standard allow to control the critical steps of sample preparation and to determine the amount of metabolite excreted [25]. The first screening analysis, which covers a wide variety of AAS (metabolites), is followed by the analysis of a second aliquot of the same specimen in case of a suspicious result in screening (confirmation).

Generally, the sample preparation for $^{13}C/^{12}C$ analysis follows the standard protocol for urinary steroids. However, the instrumental methodology requires complete conversion of the analytes to CO_2 before mass spectrometric analysis. No structural information thus can be obtained from the resulting signals. Consequently, coelutions may significantly blur the isotopic signals. Therefore, HPLC is incorporated as an additional purification step following hydrolysis [26, 27]. The obtained fractions are analyzed separately.

The mandatory conversion to CO_2 is performed online by catalytic combustion over CuO at 800–1,000°C. This conflicts with the common derivatization of steroids by silylating agents such as MSTFA. Therefore, urinary steroids are typically analyzed either in free form [27] or as acetates [14, 16, 17, 28]. Analysis of derivatized compounds requires correction of the resulting isotope ratios for the added carbons. However, the derivatization procedure may be accompanied by isotope effects which cannot be eliminated mathematically [29].

Analysis for Exogenous AAS

Steroids Explicitly Listed on WADA List

The list of prohibited substances [1] explicitly names a wide variety of exogenous AAS. Their structures are illustrated in Fig. 13.1. Detection of the misuse of these substances is preferably done using GC–MS complemented by liquid chromatography–tandem mass spectrometry (LC–MS/MS). To improve the selectivity and sensitivity, traditional GC–MS methods are accompanied by high-resolution mass spectrometry (HRMS) and/or MS/MS techniques. Special focus is given on the main and the long-term metabolites. The laboratories are obliged to test for the parent substance or metabolites with a minimum sensitivity of 10 ng/mL for anabolic agents in general and with 2 ng/mL for the metabolites

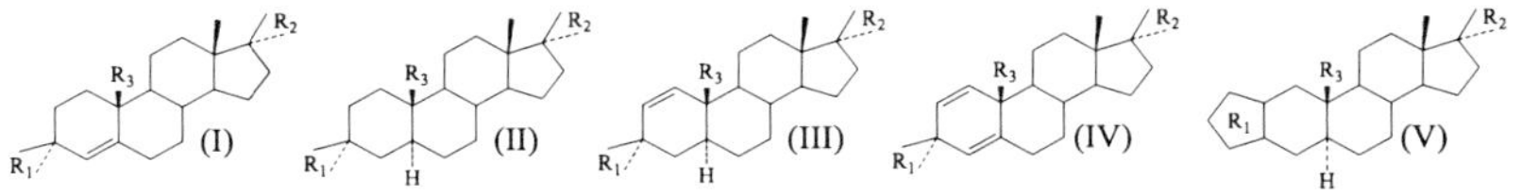

Type	R₁	R₂	R₃	Further substituents	Name WADA list
III	HO–⟨H⟩	–OH/–H	CH₃		1-Androstenediol
III	O=	=O	CH₃		1-Androstenedione
I	HO–⟨H⟩	–OH/–H	H		Bolandiol (19-norandrostenediol)
I	O=	–OH/–CH₃	CH₃	7α-CH₃	Bolasterone
IV	O=	–OH/–H	CH₃		Boldenone
IV	O=	=O	CH₃		Boldione
I	O=	–OH/–CH₃	CH₃	7β-CH₃	Calusterone
I	O=	–OH/–H	CH₃	4-Cl	Clostebol
V	N,O	–OH/–C≡CH	CH₃	delta-4	Danazol
IV	O=	–OH/–CH₃	CH₃	4-Cl	Dehydrochlormethyltestosterone
II	H-	–OH/–CH₃	CH₃	delta-2	Desoxymethyltestosterone
II	O=	–OH/–H	CH₃	2α-CH₃	Drostanolone
I	H–⟨H⟩	–OH/–C₂H₅	H		Ethylestrenol
I	O=	–OH/–CH₃	CH₃	9α-F, 11β-OH	Fluoxymesterone
IV	O=	–OH/–CH₃	CH₃	2-CHO, 11α-OH	Formebolone
V	N,N	–OH/–CH₃	CH₃		Furazabol
I	O=	–OH/–C≡CH	H	18-CH3	Gestrinone
I	O=	–OH/–H	CH₃	4-OH	4-Hydroxytestosterone
II	O=	–OH/–CH₃	CH₃		Mestanolone
II	O=	–OH/–H	CH₃	1α-CH₃	Mesterolone
III	O=	–OH/–H	CH₃	1-CH₃	Metenolone
IV	O=	–OH/–CH₃	CH₃		Metandienone
II	HO–⟨H⟩	–OH/–CH₃	CH₃	delta-5	Methandriol
II	O=	–OH/–CH₃	CH₃	2α-CH₃	Methasterone
I	O=	–OH/–CH₃	H	delta-9(10)	Methyldienolone
III	O=	–OH/–CH₃	CH₃		Methyl-1-testosterone
I	O=	–OH/–CH₃	H		Methylnortestosterone
I	O=	–OH/–CH₃	H	delta-9,11	Methyltrienolone
I	O=	–OH/–CH₃	CH₃		Methyltestosterone
I	O=	–OH/–CH₃	H	7α-CH₃	Mibolerone
I	O=	–OH/–H	H		Nandrolone
I	O=	=O	H		19-Norandrostenedione
I	O=	–OH/–C₂H₅	H	18-CH₃	Norbolethone
I	O=	–OH/–H	H	4-Cl	Norclostebol
I	O=	–OH/–CH₃	H	18-CH₃	Norethandrolone
I	O=	–OH/–H	H	4-OH	Oxabolone
II	O=	–OH/–CH₃	CH₃	2-oxa	Oxandrolone
I	O=	–OH/–CH₃	CH₃	4-OH	Oxymesterone
II	O=	–OH/–CH₃	CH₃	2=CHOH	Oxymetholone
V	HN,N	–OH/–H	CH₃		Prostanozol
IV	O=	O/–H	CH₃		Quinbolone
V	HN,N	–OH/–CH₃	CH₃		Stanozolol
III	O=	–OH/–H	CH₃	2-CH₃	Stenbolone
III	O=	–OH/–H	CH₃		1-Testosterone
I	O=	–OH/–C₂H₅	H	delta-9,11, 18-CH₃	Tetrahydrogestrinone
I	O=	–OH/–H	H	delta-9,11	Trenbolone

Fig. 13.1 Chemical structure of exogenous anabolic androgenic steroids

of metandienone (17β-methyl-5β-androst-1-ene-3α,17α-diol), methyltestosterone (17α-methyl-5β-androstane-3α,17β-diol), and stanozolol (3′-hydroxystanozolol) [30]. Criteria for substance identification as proposed by WADA [31] include the retention time and the relative abundances of at least three diagnostic ions or ion transitions compared to reference urines or reference substances. Methods for the synthesis of these reference metabolites are described by Schänzer and Donike [32].

New "Designer Steroids"

Lately, more and more products appeared on the market as "dietary supplements". They contain steroids that had never been marketed as approved drugs, mostly without proper labeling of the contents [33]. Syntheses and few data on pharmacological effects are available dated back mainly to the 1950s or 1960s. Only little knowledge exists about effects and side effects of these steroids in humans. They are only produced for the "supplement market" and are advertised as anabolic steroids or aromatase inhibitors.

The legal status of these supplements is not clear in several countries. With these "new" steroids, it is possible to circumvent the Anabolic Steroid Control Act 2004 [34]. According to this act, anabolic steroids are classified as schedule III controlled drugs and their trade as nutritional supplements is prohibited in the USA. However, these new steroids are not listed in the annex of banned steroids [34]. European legislation classifies these products as nonlicensed pharmaceuticals even if they are marketed as nutritional supplements. In most cases, the labeling of these products consists of nonapproved or fancy names of the steroids. The sources are not known but most likely Chinese pharmaceutical companies are involved. Some of the new steroids detected are advertised in their product lists on the Internet. In sports, these new steroids belong to the prohibited classes of AAS or aromatase inhibitors [1]. These steroids are not mentioned explicitly on the WADA list of prohibited substances but are covered by the wording "…and other substances with a similar chemical structure or similar biological effect(s)." The relevance of such supplements in athletes was proven in 2006 where metabolites of 6α-methylandrostenedione were found in an athlete's urine [35]. Also metabolites of androsta-1,4,6-triene-3,17-dione were already detected in doping control urines [36]. To cover the whole range of these "designer steroids," comprehensive screening tools are required. Applying mass spectrometric techniques like GC–MS or LC–MS/MS offers the possibility of unknown steroid detection [37] by monitoring common fragment ions or losses indicating the principle structure and functional groups. Especially, the precursor ion scanning option of triple–quadrupole mass analyzers is a useful tool for the detection of unknown steroids when focusing on product ions derived from common steroid structures and nuclei [38, 39].

Analysis for Endogenous AAS

The administration of AAS that are capable of being physiologically produced by the human body is also prohibited in sports. Table 13.1 summarizes the structures of the endogenous steroids listed explicitly by WADA. As these compounds and their metabolites also occur naturally in the human body-specific indicators for the detection of the exogenous administration of these steroids are required [40].

Steroid Profiling

For screening purpose, a set of urinary concentrations of several endogenous steroids or metabolites (Table 13.1) is generally determined by the GC–MS method used for

Table 13.1 Endogenous steroids listed explicitly by WADA (monitored in steroid profiling) and additionally monitored steroid profile parameters (indicated with asterisks)

Name	Type	R_1	R_2	R_3	Additional modification
Androst-5-ene-3ξ,17ξ-diol	II	–OH	–OH	–CH$_3$	delta-5
Androst-4-ene-3,17-dione	I	=O	=O	–CH$_3$	
Dihydrotestosterone	II	=O	–OH	–CH$_3$	
Dehydroepiandrosterone (DHEA)	II	–OH	=O	–CH$_3$	delta-5
Testosterone	I	=O	–OH	–CH$_3$	
5α-Androstane-3ξ,17ξ-diol	II	–OH	–OH	–CH$_3$	
5α-Androstane-3,17-dione	II	=O	=O	–CH$_3$	
17-Epi-dihydrotestosterone	II	=O	–OH	–CH$_3$	
Epitestosterone (17α-hydroxyandrost-4-ene-3-one)	I	=O	–OH	–CH$_3$	
Androsterone (3α-hydroxy-5α-androstan-17-one)	II	–OH	=O	–CH$_3$	
Etiocholanolone (3α-hydroxy-5β-androstan-17-one)	II	–OH	=O	–CH$_3$	5β-H
19-Norandrosterone (3α-hydroxy-5α-estran-17-one)	II	–OH	=O	–H	
19-Noretiocholanolone (3α-hydroxy-5β-estran-17-one)	II	–OH	=O	–H	5β-H
5β-Androstane-3ξ,17ξ-diol*	II	–OH	–OH	–CH$_3$	5β-H
5β-Androstane-3,17-dione*	II	=O	=O	–CH$_3$	5β-H
Epiandrosterone (3β-hydroxy-5α-androstan-17-one)*	II	–OH	=O	–CH$_3$	
Boldenone*	IV	=O	–OH	–CH$_3$	
17β-Hydroxy-5β-androst-1-en-3-one*	III	=O	–OH	–CH$_3$	5β-H
11β-Hydroxy-androsterone*	II	–OH	=O	–CH$_3$	11β-OH
11β-Hydroxy-etiocholanolone*	II	–OH	=O	–CH$_3$	11β-OH, 5β-H
5β-Pregnane-3α,20α-diol*	II	–OH		–CH$_3$	17β-CH(OH)CH3
5β-Pregnane-3α,17α,20α-triol*	II	–OH	–OH	–CH$_3$	17β-CH(OH)CH3

"ξ" represents "α" and/or "β" orientation
For allocation of structure types, see Fig. 13.1

the detection of steroid abuse. The method of steroid profiling was first introduced into routine doping control by Donike et al. [41] (T/E ratio). Some ratios of these steroids have been proven to be very stable [42–48]. Especially, the intraindividual variances are quite small. But also population-based reference ranges are suitable for screening purpose. Longitudinal and retrospective evaluation of steroid profiles offers a suitable basis for individual reference ranges.

The most important steroid profile parameters in doping control are the ratios of T/E, And/Etio, And/T, and Adiol/Bdiol. The administration of steroids like testosterone, its precursors like androstenediol, androstenedione, or DHEA, or metabolites, dihydrotestosterone, or epitestosterone are proven to alter one or more of the parameters of the urinary steroid profile [41, 49–55]. Consequently, monitoring the steroid profile parameters allows to screen for potential misuse.

Isotope Ratio Mass Spectrometry

The analysis of $^{13}C/^{12}C$ ratios at natural abundance levels typically is performed in a dedicated instrument known as (gas) isotope ratio mass spectrometer. As the number of applications currently is increasing dramatically, this technology often is recognized as very modern. However, the principal design has not been changed since the 1940s [56]. Basically, it is a magnetic sector field mass spectrometer where the detection is performed simultaneously for few relevant species [57]. What has been developed only recently is a diversity of peripherals allowing for rapid and precise online analysis of isotope ratios of a variety of compounds and materials. GC hyphenation has been introduced in the 1980s [58]. Commercial instrumentation based on the design of Brandt [59] is available since the early 1990s. The development is far from complete and several improvements have been introduced [60–62] recently.

References

1. World Anti-Doping Agency. The 2009 Prohibited List. Vol. 2009: World Anti-Doping Agency, 2008.
2. World Anti-Doping Agency. Adverse Analytical Findings Reported by Accredited Laboratories. Vol. 2008.
3. Schänzer W, Geyer H, Donike M. Metabolism of metandienone in man – identification and synthesis of conjugated excreted urinary metabolites, determination of excretion rates and gas-chromatographic mass-spectrometric identification of bis-hydroxylated metabolites. Journal of Steroid Biochemistry and Molecular Biology. 1991; 38:441–464.
4. Schänzer W, Opfermann G, Donike M. Metabolism of stanozolol – identification and synthesis of urinary metabolites. Journal of Steroid Biochemistry and Molecular Biology. 1990; 36:153–174.
5. Schänzer W, Horning S, Donike M. Metabolism of anabolic-steroids in humans - synthesis of 6-beta-hydroxy metabolites of 4-chloro-1,2-dehydro-17-alpha-methyltestosterone, fluoxymesterone, and metandienone. Steroids. 1995; 60:353–366.

6. Schänzer W, Horning S, Opfermann G, Donike M. Gas chromatography mass spectrometry identification of long-term excreted metabolites of the anabolic steroid 4-chloro-1,2-dehydro-17 alpha-methyltestosterone in humans. Journal of Steroid Biochemistry and Molecular Biology. 1996; 57:363–376.
7. Parr MK, Geyer H, Gütschow M, et al. New Steroids on the "Supplement" Market. Köln: 26th Cologne Workshop on Doping Analysis, 2008.
8. Sobolevsky T, Virus E, Semenistaya E, Kachala V, Kachala I, Rodchenkov G. Orastan-A: Structural Elucidation and Detection in Urine. Köln: 26th Cologne Workshop on Doping Analysis, 2008.
9. Rodchenkov G, Sobolevsky T, Sizoi V. New designer anabolic steroids from internet. In: Schänzer W, Geyer H, Gotzmann A, Mareck U, eds. Recent Advances in Doping Analysis (14). Köln: Sport und Buch Strauß, 2006:141–150.
10. Kazlauskas R. Micellaneous projects in sports drug testing at the National Measurement Institute, Australia, 2005. In: Schänzer W, Geyer H, Gotzmann A, Mareck U, eds. Recent Advances in Doping Analysis (14). Köln: Sport und Buch Strauß, 2006:129–140.
11. Schänzer W, Opfermann G, Donike M. 17-Epimerization of 17-alpha-methyl anabolic-steroids in humans – metabolism and synthesis of 17-alpha-hydroxy-17-beta-methyl steroids. Steroids. 1992; 57:537–550.
12. Kleemann A, Roth HJ. Arzneistoffgewinnung: Naturstoffe und Derivate. Stuttgart: Thieme, 1983.
13. Schänzer W. Metabolism of anabolic androgenic steroids. Clinical Chemistry. 1996; 42: 1001–1020.
14. Becchi M, Aguilera R, Farizon Y, Flament M, Casabianca H, James P. Gas chromatography/combustion/isotope-ratio mass spectrometry analysis of urinary steroids to detect misuse of testosterone in sport. Rapid Communications in Mass Spectrometry. 1994; 8:304–308.
15. Aguilera R, Hatton C, Catlin D. Detection of epitestosterone doping by isotope ratio mass spectrometry. Clinical Chemistry. 2002; 48:629–636.
16. Aguilera R, Becchi M, Casabianca H, et al. Improved method of detection of testosterone abuse by gas chromatography/combustion/isotope ratio mass spectrometry analysis of urinary steroids. Journal of Mass Spectrometry. 1996; 31:169–176.
17. Aguilera R, Becchi M, Grenot C, Casabianca H, Hatton C. Detection of testosterone misuse: comparison of two chromatographic sample preparation methods for gas chromatographic–combustion/isotope ratio mass spectrometric analysis. Journal of Chromatography B. 1996; 687:43–53.
18. Aguilera R, Chapman T, Catlin D. A rapid screening assay for measuring urinary androsterone and etiocholanolone d^{13}C values by gas chromatography/combustion/isotope ratio mass spectrometry. Rapid Communications in Mass Spectrometry. 2000; 14:2294–2299.
19. Aguilera R, Chapman T, Starcevic B, Hatton C, Catlin D. Performance characteristics of a carbon isotope ratio method for detecting doping with testosterone based on urine diols: controls and athletes with elevated testosterone/epitestosterone ratios. Clinical Chemistry. 2001; 47:292–300.
20. Vogel J. Fractionation of the Carbon Isotopes During Photosynthesis. Berlin: Springer-Verlag, 1980.
21. O'Leary M. Carbon isotope fractionation in plants. Phytochemistry. 1981; 20:553–567.
22. Donike M. N-methyl-N-trimethylsilyl-trifluoroacetamide a new silylating agent from series of silylated amides. Journal of Chromatography. 1969; 42:103–104.
23. Schänzer W. Analytik von Dopingsubstanzen – Derivatisierung. Vol. 2009: Institut für Biochemie, Deutsche Sporthochschule Köln, 2001.
24. Donike M, Zimmermann J. Preparation of trimethylsilyl, triethylsilyl and tert-butyldimethylsilyl enol ethers from ketosteroids for investigations by gas-chromatography and mass-spectrometry. Journal of Chromatography. 1980; 202:483–486.
25. Geyer H, Schänzer W, Mareck-Engelke U, Nolteernsting E, Opfermann G. Screening procedure for anabolic steroids – control of hydrolysis with deuterated androsterone glucuronide and studies with direct hydrolysis. In: Mareck-Engelke U, ed. Recent Advances in Doping Analysis (5). Köln: Sport und Buch Strauss, 1998:99–102.

26. Flenker U, Horning S, Nolteernsting E, Geyer H, Schänzer W. Measurement of $^{13}C/^{12}C$-ratios to confirm misuse of endogenous steroids. In: Schänzer W, Geyer H, Gotzmann A, Mareck-Engelke U, eds. Recent Advances in Doping Analysis (6). Köln: Sport und Buch Strauss, 1999:243–256.
27. Flenker U, Güntner U, Schänzer W. Delta C-13-values of endogenous urinary steroids. Steroids. 2008; 73:408–416.
28. Piper T, Mareck U, Geyer H, et al. Determination of C-13/C-12 ratios of endogenous urinary steroids: method validation, reference population and application to doping control purposes. Rapid Communications in Mass Spectrometry. 2008; 22:2161–2175.
29. Docherty G, Jones V, Evershed R. Practical and theoretical considerations in the gas chromatography/combustion/isotope ratio mass spectrometry d^{13}C analysis of small polyfunctional compounds. Rapid Communications in Mass Spectrometry. 2001; 15:730–738.
30. World Anti-Doping Agency. WADA Technical Document TD2009MRPL. Vol. 2009: World Anti-Doping Agency, 2008.
31. World Anti-Doping Agency. WADA Technical Document TD2003IDCR. Vol. 2009: World Anti-Doping Agency, 2004.
32. Schänzer W, Donike M. Metabolism of anabolic-steroids in man – synthesis and use of reference substances for identification of anabolic-steroid metabolites. Analytica Chimica Acta. 1993; 275:23–48.
33. Geyer H, Parr MK, Koehler K, Mareck U, Schanzer W, Thevis M. Nutritional supplements cross-contaminated and faked with doping substances. Journal of Mass Spectrometry. 2008; 43:892–902.
34. US Drug Enforcement Administration. Anabolic Steroids Control Act. Vol. 2005: US Drug Enforcement Administration, 2004.
35. Parr MK, Kazlauskas R, Schlorer N, et al. 6 alpha-Methylandrostenedione: gas chromatographic mass spectrometric detection in doping control. Rapid Communications in Mass Spectrometry. 2008; 22:321–329.
36. Parr MK, Fußhöller G, Schlörer N, et al. Metabolism of androsta-1,4,6-triene-3,17-dione and detection by gas chromatography/mass spectrometry in doping control. Rapid Communications in Mass Spectrometry. 2009; 23:207–218.
37. Thevis M, Schanzer W. Mass spectrometry in sports drug testing: Structure characterization and analytical assays. Mass Spectrometry Reviews. 2007; 26:79–107.
38. Thevis M, Geyer H, Mareck U, Schänzer W. Screening for unknown synthetic steroids in human urine by liquid chromatography–tandem mass spectrometry. Journal of Mass Spectrometry. 2005; 40:955–962.
39. Pozo OJ, Deventer K, Eenoo PV, Delbeke FT. Efficient approach for the comprehensive detection of unknown anabolic steroids and metabolites in human urine by liquid chromatography–electrospray–tandem mass spectrometry. Analytical Chemistry. 2008; 80:1709–1720.
40. World Anti-Doping Agency. WADA Technical Document TD2004EAAS. Vol. 2007: World Anti-Doping Agency, 2004.
41. Donike M, Barwald KR, Klostermann K, Schanzer W, Zimmermann J. The detection of exogenous testosterone. International Journal of Sports Medicine. 1983; 4:68.
42. Geyer H. Die gas-chromatographisch/massenspektrometrische Bestimmung von Steroidprofilen im Urin von Athleten, Institute of Biochemistry. Köln: German Sport University, 1986.
43. Mareck-Engelke U, Geyer H, Donike M. Stability of steroid profiles. In: Donike M, Geyer H, Gotzmann A, Mareck-Engelke U, Rauth S, eds. 10th Cologne Workshop on Dope Analysis. Köln: Sport und Buch Strauss, 1992:87–89.
44. Mareck-Engelke U, Geyer H, Donike M. Stability of steroid profiles (2): excretion rates from morning urines. In: Donike M, Geyer H, Gotzmann A, Mareck-Engelke U, Rauth S, eds. Recent Advances in Doping Analysis. Köln: Sport und Buch Strauss, 1993:85.
45. Mareck-Engelke U, Geyer H, Donike M. Stability of steroid profiles (4): the circadian rhythm of urinary ratios and excretion rates of endogenous steroids in female and its menstrual dependency. In: Donike M, Geyer H, Gotzmann A, Mareck-Engelke U, eds. Recent Advances in Doping Analysis (2). Köln: Sport und Buch Strauss, 1994:135.

46. Mareck-Engelke U, Geyer H, Donike M. Stability of steroid profiles (3): the circadian rhythm of urinary ratios and excretion rates of endogenous steroids in male. In: Donike M, Geyer H, Gotzmann A, Mareck-Engelke U, eds. Recent Advances in Doping Analysis (2). Köln: Sport und Buch Strauss, 1994:121.

47. Mareck-Engelke U, Geyer H, Donike M. Stability of steroid profiles (5): the annual rhythm of urinary ratios and excretion rates of endogenous steroids in female and its menstrual dependency. In: Donike M, Geyer H, Gotzmann A, Mareck-Engelke U, eds. Recent Advances in Doping Analysis (3). Köln: Sport und Buch Strauss, 1995:177.

48. Nitschke R. Steroidprofile und Ver¨anderungen biochemischer Parameter bei Hochleistungsradrennfahreren während zwei Rundfahrten, Institute of Biochemistry. Köln: German Sport University, 1996.

49. Dehennin L, Matsumoto AM. Long-term administration of testosterone enanthate to normal men: alterations of the urinary profile of androgen metabolites potentially useful for detection of testosterone misuse in sport. Journal of Steroid Biochemistry and Molecular Biology. 1993; 44:179–189.

50. Donike M, Ueki M, Kuroda Y, et al. Detection of dihydrotestosterone (DHT) doping: alterations in the steroid profile and reference ranges for DHT and its 5alpha-metabolites. Journal of Sports Medicine and Physical Fitness. 1995; 35:235–250.

51. Thevis M, Geyer H, Mareck U, Flenker U, Schanzer W. Doping-control analysis of the 5 alpha-reductase inhibitor finasteride: determination of its influence on urinary steroid profiles and detection of its major urinary metabolite. Therapeutic Drug Monitoring. 2007; 29:236–247.

52. Bowers LD. Oral dehydroepiandrosterone supplementation can increase the testosterone/epitestosterone ratio. Clinical Chemistry. 1999; 45:295–297.

53. Uralets VP, Gillette PA. Over-the-counter anabolic steroids 3-androsten-3,17-dione; 4-androsten-3 beta,17 beta-diol; and 19-nor-4-androsten-3,17-dione: excretion studies in men. Journal of Analytical Toxicology. 1999; 23:357–366.

54. Dehennin L, Ferry M, Lafarge P, Peres G, Lafarge JP. Oral administration of dehydroepiandrosterone to healthy men: alteration of the urinary androgen profile and consequences for the detection of abuse in sport by gas chromatography–mass spectrometry. Steroids. 1998; 63:80–87.

55. Geyer H, Schänzer W, Mareck-Engelke U, Donike M. Factors influencing the steroid profile. In: Donike M, Geyer H, Gotzmann A, Mareck-Engelke U, eds. Recent Advances in Doping Analysis (3). Köln: Sport und Buch Strauss, 1995:95–113.

56. De Laeter J, Kurz M. Alfred Nier and the sector field mass spectrometer. Journal of Mass Spectrometry. 2006; 41:847–854.

57. Habfast K. Advanced isotope ratio mass spectrometry I: magnetic isotope ratio mass spectrometers. In: Platzner I, ed. Modern Isotope Ratio Mass Spectrometry, Vol. 145. Chemical Analysis. Chichester: John Wiley & Sons Ltd, 1997:11–82.

58. Barrie A, Bricout J, Koziet J. Gas chromatography-stable isotope ratio analysis at natural abundance levels. Biomedical Mass Spectrometry. 1984; 11:583–588.

59. Brand W. High precision isotope ratio monitoring techniques in mass spectrometry. Journal of Mass Spectrometry. 1996; 31:225–235.

60. Flenker U, Hebestreit M, Piper T, Hülsemann F, Schänzer W. Improved performance and maintenance in gas chromatography/isotope ratio mass spectrometry by precolumn solvent removal. Analytical Chemistry. 2007; 79:4162–4168.

61. Sacks G, Zhang Y, Brenna J. Fast gas chromatography combustion isotope ratio mass spectrometry. Analytical Chemistry. 2007; 79:6348–6358.

62. Tobias H, Sacks G, Zhang Y, Brenna J. Comprehensive two-dimensional gas chromatography combustion isotope ratio mass spectrometry. Analytical Chemistry. 2008; 80:8613–8621.

Chapter 14
Problems with Growth Hormone Doping in Sports: Isoform Methods

Martin Bidlingmaier, Zida Wu, and Christian J. Strasburger

Background: GH and Its Molecular Isoforms

Human GH circulating in the bloodstream is not a homogenous, distinct substance. It is a heterogeneous mixture of molecular isoforms of this proteohormone [1]. The heterogeneity is caused on different levels [2]: Within a cluster of five similar genes on chromosome 17q, two genes, hGH-1 (or hGH-N) and hGH-2 (or hGH-V), encode for GH. Under normal conditions, the anterior pituitary releases GH-N. The other variant (GH-V) is exclusively produced by the syncytiotrophoblasts of the placenta during pregnancy [3]. Both GH-V and -N are produced as a single chain of 191 amino acids with a molecular weight of 22 kD, but with a difference in 13 amino acid residues. In addition to the major GH-N isoform with a molecular weight of 22 kD, the pituitary gland also secretes different isoforms and fragments of GH. The second most abundant isoform, 20 kD GH, is produced through alternative mRNA splicing [4] leading to omission of an internal sequence of 15 amino acids (amino acids 32–46). Twenty kilodalton GH makes up about 5–10% of the pituitary GH secretion. Biological activities of the 20 kD and the 22 kD isoform seem to be similar, although some differences have been reported with respect to their potency to modulate lipolysis and glucose metabolism. Until today, no particular stimulus of the secretion of the one or the other isoform has been identified. Therefore, it is assumed that 20 and 22 kD GH are cosecreted in a fixed ratio. In circulation, however, there seem to be differences in the half life. It has been shown that the relative proportion of "non-22 kD GH isoforms" can increase immediately post exercise [5]. Other studies, using glutathione as a reducing agent to break disulphide bonds linking GH aggregates, have provided data suggesting that the exercise-induced increase in circulating GH mainly is due to an increase in disulphide-linked dimeric isoforms of GH [6]. In addition to the two major isoforms, various other moieties of GH have been described [7], e.g., 17 kD GH and a smaller 5 kD fragment. Pituitary GH

M. Bidlingmaier (✉)
Endocrine Laboratory, Medizinische Klinik – Innenstadt,
Ludwig-Maximilians-University, Munich, Germany
e-mail: martin.bidlingmaier@med.uni-muenchen.de

E. Ghigo et al. (eds.), *Hormone Use and Abuse by Athletes*, Endocrine Updates 29,
DOI 10.1007/978-1-4419-7014-5_14, © Springer Science+Business Media, LLC 2011

extracts have been shown to also contain posttranslationally modified 22 kD GH variants such as two deaminated forms and an N-acetylated form. Other known fragments of GH are GH_{1-43} and GH_{44-191}. It is important to keep in mind that the heterogeneity of GH isoforms in circulation is not necessarily identical to the heterogeneity seen at a pituitary level [8]. This is in part due to differences in the clearance rates among isoforms [9]. Furthermore, in circulation, the molecular heterogeneity of GH is increased through the formation of hetero-, homo-dimers, and multimers of the various forms of GH. In addition, approximately 45% of the GH molecules in circulation are complexed to a high affinity growth hormone-binding protein (GHBP), which represents the extracellular domain of the GH receptor [10]. Also, a modified alpha-2-macroglobulin has been identified to serve as a low affinity but high capacity-binding protein for GH, accounting for 5–8% of complexed GH in circulation [11].

Immunoassays to Measure GH Isoforms

In clinical practice, many different commercially available or in-house immunoassays are used to measure GH. The spectrum ranges from competitive assays to sandwich type assays, and the various methods employ polyclonal antisera as well as mono-clonal antibodies, or a combination of both [12]. It has been reported by several groups that, depending on the assay used, the actual concentration of GH reported for the same sample can vary considerably. The poor agreement in results from different GH immunoassays provides problems in definition of diagnostic criteria and application of clinical guidelines [13]. Apart from differences in assay calibra-tion, the existence of various molecular isoforms of GH is discussed as one of the main factors responsible for the discrepancies: Depending on the epitope recog-nized by the respective antibodies used, each assay will translate into a signal only a certain spectrum of all GH isoforms present in a sample. Polyclonal antisera (representing a mixture of different antibodies) tend to recognize a broader spec-trum of isoforms than monoclonal antibodies (which are restricted to a single epitope), and it has been speculated that this difference explains why the dis-crepancy between the results from different assays increased when monoclonal antibody-based assays have been introduced in clinical routine in the 90s. However, for most commercially available GH immunoassays, the precise epitopes and there-fore the spectrum of isoforms recognized are unknown. International attempts have been started to reduce the variability between the different GH assays used to diag-nose GH-related diseases [14]. Such a harmonization might be desirable from a clinical point of view, but for scientists the highly specific antibodies also represent an interesting tool to develop assays specific for specific isoforms. Among the first developments into this direction was the establishment of an assay for the measure-ment of "non 22 kD GH" [15]. In this assay, 22 kD GH is first removed from the samples using a 22 kD GH-specific antibody. All isoforms remaining in the sample after this affinity extraction step are then measured by a polyclonal assay which is expected to recognize a wide spectrum of isoforms. As a more direct way to investigate GH isoforms, several assays have been developed to specifically measure the 20 kD isoform [16, 17]. This was possible only when highly specific monoclonal antibodies for 20 kD GH became available, because in view of the comparably small amount of 20 kD GH present in serum, already a minor cross-reactivity of the antibodies with 22 kD GH would have prevented the accurate quantification of the minor isoform. As mentioned above, the use of these assays has confirmed that 20 kD GH usually is cosecreted with 22 kD GH [18, 19], and that the relative proportion of 20 kD GH in circulation varies between 5 and 15% of total GH [8, 20]. Also, assays designed to specifically measure smaller fragments [21] or the placental GH variant [22] have been used in some research studies. Finally, some of the GH immunoassays specifically measure the 22 kD isoform. Examples are the Hybritech [23] and the Wallac assay, and also the "rec assays" from the differential immunoassay approach described in the next paragraph [24] belong to this category.

Detecting Changes in the Spectrum of Circulating GH Isoforms After Injection of Recombinant GH

In contrast to the wide spectrum of GH isoforms and complexes secreted by the pituitary gland and circulating in the blood stream, recombinant GH as used for therapeutic purposes and also abused to enhance performance consists of the 22 kD isoform only. Theoretically, recombinant production of other isoforms is possible, and there have been attempts to, for example, use the 20 kD isoform for treatment of GH deficiency [25]. However, no preparation is currently in clinical use or commercially available. Once recombinant 22 kD GH is injected, it binds to and activates GH receptors, thereby initiating IGF-I secretion and other known actions of GH. Furthermore, the pituitary secretion of GH molecules is suppressed through negative feedback. The latter mechanism is the rationale for the "isoform method" [26, 27] developed to detect GH doping in sports: Although it is impossible to discriminate the individual 22 kD GH molecules secreted by the pituitary gland from the molecules derived from the recombinant GH preparation, it is possible to observe a shift in the whole spectrum of GH isoforms in circulation. Because of the suppression of pituitary GH secretion [17, 19], the broad spectrum of pituitary-derived GH isoforms is no longer present in circulation, whereas the 22 kD isoform becomes predominant. To analyze this, GH immunoassays have been developed with marked differences with respect to their affinity for either pure 22 kD GH or the "pituitary derived mixture of isoforms." Measuring a serum sample by an assay preferentially recognizing the 22 kD GH isoform and by another assay recognizing a broad spectrum of GH isoforms allows to calculate a ratio between both results. This ratio – termed "rec to pit ratio" – is increased after injection of 22 kD, because the "rec-assay" result is high, whereas due to the negative feedback on pituitary GH secretion, the "pit-assay result" will be comparably low. The proof of principle for this method has been demonstrated using 40 blinded samples, half of them taken after stimulation of endogenous GH secretion, the other half taken after injection of recombinant GH [28]. The absolute GH concentrations in these samples were matched in both groups and did not allow the analyzing laboratory to draw any conclusion as to the origin of the GH molecules. However, measuring the samples by a "rec-assay" and a "pit-assay" and calculation of the rec/pit ratio in this study allowed correct classification of all samples, because these samples all had a clearly elevated ratio. The concept was evaluated in a larger series of samples [27], and it could also be demonstrated that – although during exercise 22 kD GH increases slightly more than the other isoforms, after exercise the other isoforms tend to become somewhat more predominant – the corresponding changes in the rec/pit ratio are only marginal and would not compromise the use of the test in an antidoping setting [5, 29]. However, another problem had to be solved before the principle could be used for antidoping purposes: According to the world antidoping code and the international standards for WADA-accredited laboratories, an independent test is required to confirm any positive case in doping controls (also called "adverse analytical finding"). For immunoassays, "independent tests" means that antibodies recognizing independent epitopes have to be used. Accordingly, two independent sets of "rec"- and "pit"-assays were developed [27]. When applied to the same samples, the rec/pit ratios obtained by both assay combinations revealed similar results, supporting the use of one assay combination for initial screening of samples and the other assay combination for independent confirmation. Both assay combinations – based on in-house research reagents – were evaluated during the Athens (2004) and Torino (2006) Olympic games [30]. No adverse analytical findings were reported during these events. This might indicate that athletes were not taking hGH, or – probably more likely – that GH is used during training rather than competition. However, it was also obvious that the "in-house version" of the assays, which was utilizing non-routine research reagents and microtiter plates coated on site, worsened performance in terms of sensitivity and robustness. The comparably high sensitivity of 0.1 µg/L initially reported could not be routinely maintained after transfer of reagents and operating instructions to antidoping laboratories. Therefore, and to allow a widespread utilization of the test method, it was necessary to develop a more robust, sensitive, and standardized format of the test, which was achieved by transfer to a chemiluminescence-coated tube format and production of reagents and kits on a professional ISO certified level. This improved format of the test kits was thoroughly validated [24], and larger series of samples from males and females not treated with GH allowed establishment of normal ranges for the ratios. Furthermore, in an application study it could be shown that the window of opportunity for detection of a previous single injection of recombinant GH was up to 36 h in some individuals. However, rate of detection was best during the first 24 h after injection and – as expected – was better after application of a higher dose. Interestingly, the window of opportunity was significantly longer in females compared to males [24].

During the Beijing Olympic Games in Summer 2008, the differential immunoassays were first used officially in the certified format to analyze about 500 samples. Not really to the surprise of the experts, no positive test result was reported. It is an obvious problem with this method that the detection is possible only shortly after the injection of the drug – since the isoform approach is based on the direct measurement of hGH, the window of opportunity for detection is determined by the short half-life of rhGH in circulation. As a consequence, the differential immunoassay approach can be expected to be most valuable in an out-of-competition setting, when unannounced controls are performed. Full implementation of the isoform assays in WADA-accredited laboratories as well as substantial increases in the number of blood samples taken during doping controls worldwide remain the challenges for the next years to increase the chance to catch the cheaters.

Future Directions

An interesting finding when characterizing the epitopes for the antibodies involved in the differential immunoassays was that the detection antibody in all four assays has no cross-reactivity with 20 kD GH [24]. The principle of the differential immunoassays – although based on changes in GH isoform spectrum – apparently works without recognition of the second most abundant pituitary GH isoform. This opens the field for the use of assays specific for 20 kD GH as another independent confirmation of the abuse of recombinant GH: As mentioned above, it has been demonstrated that the 20 kD isoform is suppressed after application of recombinant 22 kD GH [19]. A problem with a doping test based on the "disappearance of 20 kD GH" in circulation obviously is the very low concentration of 20 D GH already seen in many subjects not treated with recombinant 22 kD GH. Of course, also for a test based on 20 kD GH, it would be required to also measure 22 kD as a reference. This could allow demonstrating that the abundance of the 20 kD isoform is lower than expected in view of a certain level of 22 kD GH. Several groups have started developing more sensitive assays selectively measuring 20 kD GH.

Other developments include the analysis of GH isoforms by methods other than immunoassays. Promising results have been published by groups using plasmon surface resonance analysis [31], 2D gel electrophoresis to visualize the isoforms present in a sample [32], and also mass spectrometry to identify GH isoforms [33]. Sensitivity is a challenging point for all methods. Until today, isoform analysis by any method usually requires the use of antibodies from immunoaffinity enrichment of the analyte. However, it can be expected that a broader spectrum of methods based on the concept of isoform recognition in the future will help to catch cheating athletes abusing GH [34].

References

1. Baumann G. Growth hormone heterogeneity: Genes, isohormones, variants, and binding proteins. Endocr Rev. 1991;12:424–49
2. Hirt H, Kimelman J, Birnbaum MJ, Chen EY, Seeburg PH, Eberhardt NL, Barta A. The human growth hormone gene locus: Structure, evolution, and allelic variations. DNA. 1987;6:59–70

3. Igout A, Van Beeumen J, Frankenne F, Scippo ML, Devreese B, Hennen G. Purification and biochemical characterization of recombinant human placental growth hormone produced in *Escherichia coli*. Biochem J. 1993;295:719–24

4. Cooke NE, Ray J, Watson MA, Estes PA, Kuo BA, Liebhaber SA. Human growth hormone gene and the highly homologous growth hormone variant gene display different splicing patterns. J Clin Invest. 1988;82:270–5

5. Wallace JD, Cuneo RC, Bidlingmaier M, Lundberg PA, Carlsson L, Boguszewski CL, Hay J, Healy ML, Napoli R, Dall R, Rosen T, Strasburger CJ. The response of molecular isoforms of growth hormone to acute exercise in trained adult males. J Clin Endocrinol Metab. 2001;86:200–6

6. Nindl BC. Exercise modulation of growth hormone isoforms: Current knowledge and future directions for the exercise endocrinologist. Br J Sports Med. 2007;41:346–8; discussion 348

7. Baumann G. Growth hormone heterogeneity in human pituitary and plasma. Horm Res. 1999;51:2–6

8. Popii V, Baumann G. Laboratory measurement of growth hormone. Clin Chim Acta. 2004; 350:1–16

9. Baumann G, Stolar MW, Buchanan TA. The metabolic clearance, distribution, and degradation of dimeric and monomeric growth hormone (GH): Implications for the pattern of circulating GH forms. Endocrinology. 1986;119:1497–501

10. Baumann G, Amburn K, Shaw MA. The circulating growth hormone (GH)-binding protein complex: A major constituent of plasma GH in man. Endocrinology. 1988;122:976–84

11. Kratzsch J, Selisko T, Birkenmeier G. Identification of transformed alpha 2-macroglobulin as a growth hormone-binding protein in human blood. J Clin Endocrinol Metab. 1995;80: 585–90

12. Bidlingmaier M, Freda PU. Measurement of human growth hormone by immunoassays: Current status, unsolved problems and clinical consequences. Growth Horm IGF Res. 2010; 20:19–25

13. Pokrajac A, Wark G, Ellis AR, Wear J, Wieringa GE, Trainer PJ. Variation in GH and IGF-I assays limits the applicability of international consensus criteria to local practice. Clin Endocrinol (Oxf). 2007;67:65–70

14. Wieringa GE, Trainer PJ. Commentary: Harmonizing growth hormone measurements: Learning lessons for the future. J Clin Endocrinol Metab. 2007;92:2874–5

15. Boguszewski CL, Hynsjo L, Johannsson G, Bengtsson BA, Carlsson LM. 22-kD growth hormone exclusion assay: A new approach to measurement of non-22-kD growth hormone isoforms in human blood. Eur J Endocrinol. 1996;135:573–82

16. Wada M, Uchida H, Ikeda M, Tsunekawa B, Naito N, Banba S, Tanaka E, Hashimoto Y, Honjo M. The 20-kilodalton (kDa) human growth hormone (hGH) differs from the 22-kDa hGH in the complex formation with cell surface hGH receptor and hGH-binding protein circulating in human plasma. Mol Endocrinol. 1998;12:146–56

17. Keller A, Wu Z, Kratzsch J, Keller E, Blum WF, Kniess A, Preiss R, Teichert J, Strasburger CJ, Bidlingmaier M. Pharmacokinetics and pharmacodynamics of GH: Dependence on route and dosage of administration. Eur J Endocrinol. 2007;156:647–53

18. Ishikawa M, Yokoya S, Tachibana K, Hasegawa Y, Yasuda T, Tokuhiro E, Hashimoto Y, Tanaka T. Serum levels of 20-kilodalton human growth hormone (GH) are parallel those of 22-kilodalton human GH in normal and short children. J Clin Endocrinol Metab. 1999;84:98–104

19. Leung KC, Howe C, Gui LY, Trout G, Veldhuis JD, Ho KK. Physiological and pharmacological regulation of 20-kDa growth hormone. Am J Physiol Endocrinol Metab. 2002;283: E836–43

20. Tsushima T, Katoh Y, Miyachi Y, Chihara K, Teramoto A, Irie M, Hashimoto Y. Serum concentration of 20K human growth hormone (20K hGH) measured by a specific enzyme-linked immunosorbent assay. Study Group of 20K hGH. J Clin Endocrinol Metab. 1999;84:317–22

21. Sinha YN, Jacobsen BP. Human growth hormone (hGH)-(44-191), a reportedly diabetogenic fragment of hGH, circulates in human blood: Measurement by radioimmunoassay. J Clin Endocrinol Metab. 1994;78:1411–8
22. Wu Z, Bidlingmaier M, Friess SC, Kirk SE, Buchinger P, Schiessl B, Strasburger CJ. A new nonisotopic, highly sensitive assay for the measurement of human placental growth hormone: Development and clinical implications. J Clin Endocrinol Metab. 2003;88:804–11
23. Celniker AC, Chen AB, Wert RM, Jr., Sherman BM. Variability in the quantitation of circulating growth hormone using commercial immunoassays. J Clin Endocrinol Metab. 1989;68: 469–76
24. Bidlingmaier M, Suhr J, Ernst A, Wu Z, Keller A, Strasburger CJ, Bergmann A. High-sensitivity chemiluminescence immunoassays for detection of growth hormone doping in sports. Clin Chem. 2009;55:445–53
25. Hayakawa M, Shimazaki Y, Tsushima T, Kato Y, Takano K, Chihara K, Shimatsu A, Irie M. Metabolic effects of 20-kilodalton human growth hormone (20K-hGH) for adults with growth hormone deficiency: Results of an exploratory uncontrolled multicenter clinical trial of 20K-hGH. J Clin Endocrinol Metab. 2004;89:1562–71
26. Bidlingmaier M, Strasburger CJ. Technology insight: Detecting growth hormone abuse in athletes. Nat Clin Pract Endocrinol Metab. 2007;3:769–77
27. Bidlingmaier M, Wu Z, Strasburger CJ. Test method: GH. Baillieres Best Pract Res Clin Endocrinol Metab. 2000;14:99–109
28. Wu Z, Bidlingmaier M, Dall R, Strasburger CJ. Detection of doping with human growth hormone. Lancet. 1999;353:895
29. Wallace JD, Cuneo RC, Bidlingmaier M, Lundberg PA, Carlsson L, Boguszewski CL, Hay J, Boroujerdi M, Cittadini A, Dall R, Rosen T, Strasburger CJ. Changes in non-22-kilodalton (kDa) isoforms of growth hormone (GH) after administration of 22-kDa recombinant human GH in trained adult males. J Clin Endocrinol Metab. 2001;86:1731–7
30. Saugy M, Robinson N, Saudan C, Baume N, Avois L, Mangin P. Human growth hormone doping in sport. Br J Sports Med. 2006;40 Suppl 1:i35–9
31. Gutierrez-Gallego R, Bosch J, Such-Sanmartin G, Segura J. Surface plasmon resonance immuno assays – A perspective. Growth Horm IGF Res. 2009;19:388–98
32. Kohler M, Puschel K, Sakharov D, Tonevitskiy A, Schanzer W, Thevis M. Detection of recombinant growth hormone in human plasma by a 2-D PAGE method. Electrophoresis. 2008;29:4495–502
33. Kohler M, Thomas A, Puschel K, Schanzer W, Thevis M. Identification of human pituitary growth hormone variants by mass spectrometry. J Proteome Res. 2009;8:1071–6
34. Segura J, Gutierrez-Gallego R, Ventura R, Pascual JA, Bosch J, Such-Sanmartin G, Nikolovski Z, Pinyot A, Pichini S. Growth hormone in sport: Beyond Beijing 2008. Ther Drug Monit. 2009;31:3–13

Chapter 15
Detection of Growth Hormone Doping in Sport Using Growth Hormone-Responsive Markers

Anne E. Nelson and Ken K.Y. Ho

Introduction

Developing a robust test for detecting a naturally occurring polypeptide such as growth hormone (GH) has been a challenge. There is anecdotal evidence for widespread abuse of GH in sport, which is often used together with other banned substances such as anabolic steroids, despite being banned by the World Anti-Doping Agency (WADA) [1]. One approach for the detection of GH is based on the measurement of serum GH-responsive markers, such as insulin-like growth factor (IGF) axis and collagen peptides. This approach should extend the window of opportunity of detection of GH and also has the potential to detect abuse with other forms of GH and GH secretagogues. There is also evidence that the sensitivity of the markers to GH may be enhanced by co-administration of testosterone [2]. The major determinants of variability for IGF-I and the collagen markers are age and gender, therefore a test based on these markers must take age into account for men and women [3]. Extensive data are now available from both administration studies and studies of the variability of the markers, which validate the GH-responsive markers approach, and implementation is now largely dependent on establishing an assured supply of standardized assays.

Abuse of Growth Hormone and Challenges in Developing a Robust Test

The abuse of GH by athletes is probably due to the immense pressure to perform in sport and there is anecdotal evidence that GH is widely abused, as indicated by the number of Web site hits for GH supply and by customs and police drugs seizures.

K.K.Y. Ho (✉)
Pituitary Research Unit, Department of Endocrinology, Garvan Institute of Medical Research
(AN, KH), St. Vincent's Hospital (KH), Sydney, NSW 2010, Australia
e-mail: k.ho@garvan.org.au

E. Ghigo et al. (eds.), *Hormone Use and Abuse by Athletes*, Endocrine Updates 29,
DOI 10.1007/978-1-4419-7014-5_15, © Springer Science+Business Media, LLC 2011

In a frequently cited survey, 98% of athletes said they would take a performance-enhancing substance that would guarantee an Olympic medal if they could not be caught, and 50% also replied yes when asked if they would take the drug with a guarantee they would not get caught and they won every competition for the next 5 years, even if they then died from its adverse effects [4]. The abuse of GH may start at young ages, with an early survey reporting abuse of GH by 5% of tenth grade boys in the USA, more than half using GH in conjunction with steroids [5]. In a 2006 survey of college athletes in the USA, 1.2% of the athletes reported using GH in the past 12 months [6]. Doses used by athletes are estimated to range from 3 to 8 mg daily for 3–4 days per week, often in combination with other doping agents [7], resulting in average daily doses of 1–2 mg GH, approximately two to three times the daily endogenous pituitary secretion. "Polypharmacy" is widely practiced, with GH reportedly used in particular with anabolic steroids. The use of GH (1–10 mg/day) with insulin and anabolic androgenic steroids (AASs) was reported by 25% of AAS users in a Web-based survey [8]. The AAS abusers typically "stack" with several AASs, with 60% of those surveyed using >1,000 mg AAS/week and a typical "complex cycle" consisting of high doses for a long period: 3,500 mg AAS/week together with 2 mg/day GH for 20 weeks [8]. Use of GH together with anabolic steroids was reported by 5% of the steroid users in another Web-based survey of weightlifters and body builders [9].

Most current tests for detecting doping use urine, which until recently was the only body fluid available for sports doping testing and compared to a blood sample, is easily obtained and in relatively large volumes. Urinary testing for GH is unlikely to be successful, however, since the urinary GH concentration is very low, at approximately 0.1–1% that in blood and is variable, with much of the variability not accounted for by the variations in serum GH [10, 11]. Although urinary GH concentration increases after administration of exogenous GH, increases can also occur following exercise [12]. Recombinant human 22 kDa GH available commercially has the identical amino acid sequence to the 22 kDa GH isoform secreted endogenously by the pituitary gland and GH administered by doping athletes cannot be distinguished from endogenous GH by current analytical methods. Although differences in glycosylation patterns have been used to distinguish between exogenous recombinant hormone and endogenously secreted hormone as the basis for a test for erythropoietin [13], this is not currently feasible for GH, which does not have N-linked glycosylation sites in the 1–191 sequence.

Direct measurement of total circulating GH cannot be used for a robust GH test due to the widely fluctuating physiological GH concentrations, in particular in response to exercise. GH has a short half-life of 15–20 min in the circulation and exogenous GH administered by injection disappears rapidly from the circulation [14]. Circulating physiological concentrations of GH vary widely, since GH is secreted from the pituitary in a pulsatile manner and is regulated by several factors, including sleep, exercise, stress, and food intake [15]. Exercise is a major stimulus to GH secretion and plasma concentrations can increase up to tenfold, with the increases in GH dependent on the duration, intensity, and nature of the exercise, as reviewed [16]. Therefore, increases in circulating GH are not specific for exogenous GH administration.

Physiological Basis for GH-Responsive Marker Approach

The physiological effects of GH that result in increased circulating concentrations of proteins, with a longer half-life and a more stable serum concentration than GH, form the basis of the GH-responsive marker approach to a GH doping test. GH stimulates production of IGF-I, which mediates many of the anabolic actions of GH, both by the liver, which is the main source of circulating IGF-I, and in other tissues. GH also stimulates the hepatic production of IGF-binding protein-3 (IGFBP-3) and the acid labile subunit (ALS) which form a circulating ternary complex with IGF-I [17, 18]. In response to GH, therefore, the serum concentrations of these IGF axis proteins increase. GH also stimulates bone and connective tissue turnover resulting in increased concentrations of specific collagen peptides related to collagen synthesis and degradation, both directly and via IGF-I [19]. These collagen peptides include the marker of bone formation: N-terminal propeptide of type I procollagen (PINP), the marker of bone resorption: C-terminal telopeptide of type I collagen (ICTP) and the marker of connective tissue synthesis: N-terminal propeptide of type III procollagen (abbreviated as PIIINP or PIIIP, referring to measurements made using different assays) [20]. The half-lives of the IGF axis proteins and collagen markers, which range from 90 to >500 h [21], are considerably longer than that of GH.

The GH-responsive markers approach was pioneered by the collaborative GH-2000 group that evaluated serum IGF axis makers: IGF-I, IGFBP-1, IGFBP-2, IGFBP-3, and ALS, and serum markers of bone and connective tissue turnover: osteocalcin, bone-specific alkaline phosphatase, C-terminal propeptide of type I collagen (PICP), ICTP, and PIIIP [22]. Studies were performed to determine the effect of exercise on these markers. Although acute exercise transiently increased IGF-I, IGFBP-3, and ALS, the increases were much smaller than those in response to GH administration alone [23]. The same was true for osteocalcin, PICP, ICTP, and PIIIP, the responses of which were greater and more prolonged following GH than after acute exercise [24].

Demographic Factors Influencing the GH-Responsive Markers

The application of the GH-responsive markers approach to a doping test requires extensive normative data in elite athletes to identify the factors influencing their levels in blood and establish normal reference ranges. In a large cross-sectional study of IGF-I, IGFBP-3, ALS, PINP, ICTP, and PIIINP in over 1,000 elite athletes from 12 countries representing four major ethnic groups, we have reported that age and gender were the major determinants of variability for IGF-I and the collagen peptides [3]. There was a significant negative correlation between age and all these GH-responsive markers, similarly to the correlation seen in the general population [25, 26] and age was the major contributor to variability especially for the collagen peptides (Fig. 15.1). To examine the effect of age on the markers in young athletes, we extended the study in athletes aged 12–18 years (32 girls and 24 boys), who were participating at the elite level in diving, gymnastics, swimming or athletics (Fig. 15.1). The concentration of the IGF axis markers (IGF-I, IGFBP-3, and ALS) increased in early adolescence to a late pubertal peak, then decreased sharply after

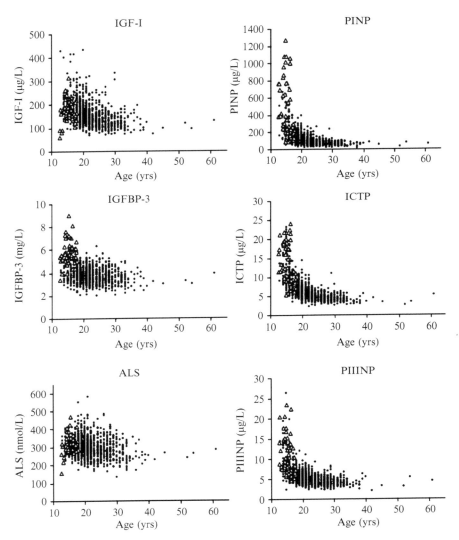

Fig. 15.1 Effect of age on IGF axis and collagen markers in young elite athletes and large cross-sectional elite athlete cohort. The measurements are plotted against age for IGF-I, IGFBP-3, and ALS (*left panel*), and PINP, ICTP, and PIIINP (*right panel*) for the young elite athletes (*triangles*) and for the large cross-sectional elite athlete cohort (*filled circle*). Adapted from [3], copyright 2006, The Endocrine Society

puberty, similarly to the changes observed in adolescents in the general population [25]. The collagen markers PINP, ICTP, and PIIINP were all markedly elevated in early adolescence in elite athletes, particularly for PINP and the subsequent rapid decrease with age was again consistent with changes in adolescence in the general population [26, 27].

There were significant differences in the markers between men and women in our large cross-sectional study of elite athletes [3]. The serum IGF markers were all higher in women and the collagen markers were higher in men; however, the contribution of gender to the variability was smaller than that of age except for IGFBP-3 and ALS (Fig. 15.2). The contributions of BMI and sport type were both modest compared with those of age and gender (Fig. 15.2). For IGF-I, PINP, and ICTP, there were no significant differences between ethnic groups following adjustment for age, gender, and BMI, whereas for IGFBP-3, ALS, and PIIINP, there were significant differences. IGFBP-3 was higher in Caucasians than in Asians and Africans and lower in Africans compared to each of the other groups. ALS was higher in Caucasians than in Asians and Africans and lower in Africans compared to each of the other groups. PIIINP was higher in Asians than in Caucasians. In multiple regression analysis, the contribution of ethnicity to the variation in IGF axis and bone turnover markers was small ($\leq 2\%$ of total variation, equivalent to $<6\%$ of the attributable variation), except for IGFBP-3 and ALS (Fig. 15.2).

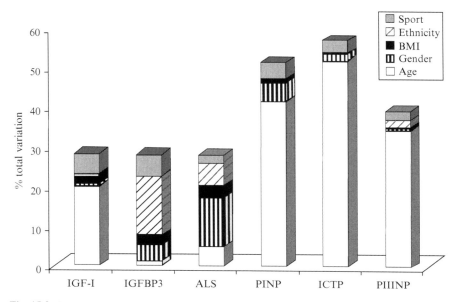

Fig. 15.2 Multiple regression analysis for sporting type analysis. The contribution of age, gender, BMI, ethnicity, and sporting type to the total variation is shown for each marker, for the analysis of 995 athletes from 7 sporting groups. Reproduced from [3], copyright 2006, The Endocrine Society

Therefore, this study of elite athletes in the out-of-competition setting indicated that a test based on IGF-I and the collagen markers must take age into account for men and women, and that ethnicity was unlikely to be a confounder for IGF-I and the collagen markers [3]. Our findings on the influence of age, gender, BMI, and sport type have also been confirmed in a study of mostly Caucasian elite athletes in the post-competition setting [28], which also concluded that sport category was not a significant predictor compared to age and gender. In the post-competition setting, some significant differences in IGF-I and PIIIP have been observed between ethnic groups; however, most observations lay below the upper 99% prediction limits derived from white European athletes. The minor differences between ethnic groups had no significant impact on the GH-2000 detection method to detect GH abuse based on IGF-I and PIIIP [29].

Variability of the GH-Responsive Markers Within Subjects

The utility of the IGF axis and collagen markers for a GH doping test in sport also depends on their stability and reproducibility. Examination of short-term variability over 2–3 weeks in our cohort of over 1,000 elite athletes showed that the within-subject variance accounted for 32–36% of the total variance in the IGF axis markers and 4–13% in the collagen markers [30]. The within-subject coefficient of variation ranged from 11 to 21% for the IGF axis markers, and from 13 to 15% for the collagen markers. Individuals with initial extreme measured values tended to regress toward the population mean in subsequent repeated measurements for each marker. A Bayesian model was developed to estimate the long-term probable value for each marker where a single measurement is available [30]. Statistical modeling, such as the Bayesian approach, therefore, may enhance the reliability of GH doping tests based on the use of these markers. Further data on longer-term within-subject variability, which has been addressed by the GH-2000 group [22], is also required.

The effect of pre-analytical storage conditions on measurements of IGF-I and PIIIP has been studied in order to determine the handling conditions that minimize the pre-analytical variability [31]. Storage temperature or timing of centrifugation did not appear to affect IGF-I concentration; however, concentrations of PIIIP changed when samples were stored at room temperature. The results indicated that while the optimum collection method is immediate centrifugation and storage at −80°C, acceptable handling would be storage of samples at 4°C for up to 5 days.

Changes in GH-Responsive Markers Following GH Administration

The changes in GH-responsive markers following administration of GH for 4 weeks was examined by the GH-2000 group in a randomized double-blind placebo-controlled study in 99 young athletically trained men and women, using two doses of GH: 0.33 mg/kg/day and 0.67 mg/kg/day. The IGF axis proteins IGF-I, IGFBP-3, and ALS all increased in response to GH, with the greatest response in IGF-I. Men were significantly more responsive than women. All IGF proteins returned to baseline within a few days of cessation of treatment, except for IGF-I which was elevated for longer in men [32]. All the markers of bone and connective tissue turnover increased in response to GH, with ICTP and PIIIP exhibiting the greatest responses and peak increments greater in men than in women. Osteocalcin, ICTP and PIIIP remained significantly elevated for up to 8 weeks after cessation of treatment, which clearly indicated the potential for a longer time window of detection using these markers [33]. Other placebo-controlled administration studies have also shown the potential for IGF axis and collagen peptides as markers of GH administration [34, 35]. An evaluation of IGFBP-4 and -5 has indicated that they will not be useful as IGF-I independent markers [36].

A double-blind placebo-controlled study of GH administration investigating the influence of gender and testosterone, has been undertaken by our group in 96 recreational athletes, aged 18–40 years [2]. GH induced significant increases in IGF axis and collagen markers which were greater in men than women. IGF-I showed the greatest increase of the IGF axis markers and PIIINP the greatest increase of the collagen markers (Fig. 15.3). The increases in collagen markers have a different time course to the IGF markers, with a slower increase and decrease, and may extend the window of detection in both sexes up to 6 weeks from cessation of treatment. This suggests that using both IGF-I and a collagen marker may provide the greatest discriminatory power for a doping test both during GH administration and withdrawal.

The different pharmacodynamic profiles of the IGF axis and collagen markers indicated by these results provide further support that a GH doping test based on the GH-responsive markers should not rely on a single marker but should use a combination of markers. Studies with extended wash out periods have shown the prolonged elevation of collagen markers after cessation of GH administration [2, 32–34], indicating the benefits of using a combination of several markers to detect GH doping both during active administration and during washout. Combinations of IGF-I, IGFBP-3, PIIINP, and ICTP have been proposed [34, 35, 37]. Our cross-sectional study also showed that no individuals had extreme values (outside the 99% reference interval) both for IGF-I and for the collagen markers in the same sample, which confirms that the use of IGF-I and a collagen marker will increase the specificity of the test [3].

Algorithms based on IGF-I and PIIINP show promise in discriminating GH-treated from placebo-treated subjects, with low false-positive rates in particular when sex-specific algorithms including age are used to account for the effects of age and gender on these markers [34, 37, 38]. Our recent GH administration study has highlighted the potential of IGF-I, PIIINP, and ICTP in combination as promising discriminators of GH administration against our reference population of elite athletes, both during treatment and for up to several weeks following treatment, due to the longer time course of the collagen marker responses (unpublished results).

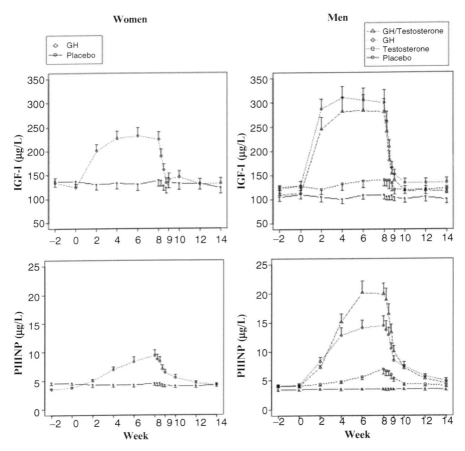

Fig. 15.3 Responses of IGF-I and PIIINP to GH and testosterone in a double-blind placebo-controlled study in 96 young recreational athletes. Serum concentrations of IGF-I (µg/l) and PIIINP (µg/l), in women and in men, before treatment (weeks −2, 0), during treatment (weeks 2, 4, 6, 8), and during the washout period (corresponding to 1, 2, 4, and 7 days, then 2, 4, and 6 weeks after the last GH/placebo injection). Data shown as mean ± SEM for each treatment group. Adapted from [2], copyright 2006, The Endocrine Society

Effects of Other Performance-Enhancing Substances and Sports Injury

A robust test for GH must also take into account the possible confounding effects of multiple performance-enhancing substances that are used by athletes practicing polypharmacy. We investigated the effect of administration of recombinant human erythropoietin (r-HuEPO) on GH-responsive markers in young male recreational athletes and found no significant treatment effect compared to baseline on IGF-I, IGFBP-3, ALS, PINP, ICTP, or PIIINP [39]. Therefore, use of r-HuEPO by athletes should not affect the validity of a test using these IGF axis and collagen markers.

The effect of testosterone on GH-responsive markers was investigated in our double-blind placebo-controlled study of 96 young recreational athletes [2]. Testosterone alone did not affect IGF-I, IGFBP-3, or ALS and increased PINP, ICTP, and PIIINP modestly. Co-administration of testosterone in men did not affect the sensitivity of these markers for detection of GH, except for PIIINP which showed an increased response (Fig. 15.3).

The effect of injury on the GH-responsive markers has also been investigated, since distinct changes in serum biochemical bone markers due to bone remodeling and collagen III synthesis in fracture healing occur following lower limb fractures [40, 41]. A longitudinal observational study in elite and amateur athletes following injury has shown no change in IGF-I, but a rise in the concentration of PIIIP that varied according injury type (soft tissue or bony injury) and severity [42]. The rise in PIIIP, however, had a trivial effect on the GH-2000 discriminant function score and was not sufficient to invalidate the GH-2000 detection method.

Implementation of a Test Based on GH-Responsive Markers

Extensive data is now available that validates the use of the GH-responsive markers; however, implementation of doping test based on this approach is dependent on the availability of assays for the measurement of the markers, that meet the requirements of WADA. The GH-responsive markers are all serum proteins, which are measured by immunoassay. For each peptide or protein measured by immunoassay, at least two independent assays must be developed, since the confirmation assay is required to use a different antibody that recognizes a different epitope of the peptide, than that used for the screening assay [43]. Development of standardized assays for the GH-responsive markers is required with assured, continuing supply of critical reagents such as the antibodies, and establishment of normative ranges using these standardized assays, before this approach can be implemented.

Summary and Future Directions

In summary, implementation of the GH-responsive marker approach will extend the time window of detection of GH. This method also has the potential to detect abuse of other agents, such as other forms of GH, GH secretagogues and IGF-I. The main hurdles to be overcome for the implementation of the markers approach as a doping test are technical and logistic issues, in particular those relating to ensuring availability to testing laboratories of standardized assays with assured supplies of antibodies.

Future directions may include the use of other platforms for the measurement of the GH-responsive markers. New immunoassay platforms, including multiplexed particle-based flow cytometric assays, such as the Luminex system [44] represent technical advances that will enhance efficiency and sensitivity. Mass spectrometry methods may also be applied to quantification of GH-responsive markers. Quantification of IGF-I and IGFBP-3 in human serum by liquid chromatography-tandem mass spectrometry (LC-MS/MS) using synthetic stable-isotope-labeled peptides as internal standards [45] and a mass-spectrometry-based assay for rat PINP [46] have been described.

The use of an "athlete's passport" that documents measurements of biological parameters over time has been proposed to assist in detection of banned substances, as recently described for erythropoietin [47]. The athlete would take a baseline test for the passport that would provide reference levels for the individual. The passport would thus enable detection of abnormal levels that differ to the baseline for that athlete due to banned substances or methods, rather than comparing levels to normative ranges alone. This has the potential to increase the sensitivity of methods, particularly those based on biomakers such as the GH-responsive marker approach.

In conclusion, robust tests should be available based on GH-responsive markers to detect GH and enforce the ban on its abuse. This approach will extend the time window of detection of GH.

Acknowledgments Research by the authors has been supported by the World Anti-Doping Agency and by the Australian Government through the *Anti-Doping Research Program* (ADRP) of the Department of Communications, Information Technology and the Arts.

References

1. Nelson AE, Ho KK. A robust test for growth hormone doping--present status and future prospects. Asian J Androl. 2008;10(3):416–25.
2. Nelson AE, Meinhardt U, Hansen JL, et al. Pharmacodynamics of growth hormone abuse bio-markers and the influence of gender and testosterone: a randomized double-blind placebo-controlled study in young recreational athletes. J Clin Endocrinol Metab. 2008;93(6):2213–22.
3. Nelson AE, Howe CJ, Nguyen TV, et al. Influence of demographic factors and sport type on growth hormone-responsive markers in elite athletes. J Clin Endocrinol Metab. 2006;91(11):4424–32.
4. Bamberger M, Yaeger D. Over the edge: special report. Sports Illus. 1997;86:64.
5. Rickert VI, Pawlak-Morello C, Sheppard V, Jay MS. Human growth hormone: a new substance of abuse among adolescents? Clin Pediatr (Phila). 1992;31(12):723–6.
6. National Collegiate Athletic Association. NCAA study of substance use of college student-athletes. 2006 (Accessed 2008: www.ncaa.org/library/research/substance_use_habits/2006/2006_substance_use_report.pdf.).
7. Saugy M, Robinson N, Saudan C, Baume N, Avois L, Mangin P. Human growth hormone doping in sport. Br J Sports Med. 2006;40(Suppl 1):i35–9.
8. Parkinson AB, Evans NA. Anabolic androgenic steroids: a survey of 500 users. Med Sci Sports Exerc. 2006;38(4):644–51.
9. Perry PJ, Lund BC, Deninger MJ, Kutscher EC, Schneider J. Anabolic steroid use in weightlifters and bodybuilders: an internet survey of drug utilization. Clin J Sport Med. 2005;15(5):326–30.
10. Weissberger AJ, Ho KY, Stuart MC. Quantification of urinary growth hormone (GH) excretion by centrifugal ultrafiltration and radioimmunoassay: appraisal of the relationship between 24 h urinary GH and mean 24 h serum GH levels in normal and abnormal states of GH secretion. Clin Endocrinol (Oxf). 1989;30(6):687–98.

11. Flanagan DE, Taylor MC, Parfitt V, Mardell R, Wood PJ, Leatherdale BA. Urinary growth hormone following exercise to assess growth hormone production in adults. Clin Endocrinol (Oxf). 1997;46(4):425–9.
12. Saugy M, Cardis C, Schweizer C, Veuthey JL, Rivier L. Detection of human growth hormone doping in urine: out of competition tests are necessary. J Chromatogr B Biomed Appl. 1996; 687(1):201–11.
13. Kazlauskas R, Howe C, Trout G. Strategies for rhEPO detection in sport. Clin J Sport Med. 2002;12(4):229–35.
14. Holl RW, Schwarz U, Schauwecker P, Benz R, Veldhuis JD, Heinze E. Diurnal variation in the elimination rate of human growth hormone (GH): the half-life of serum GH is prolonged in the evening, and affected by the source of the hormone, as well as by body size and serum estradiol. J Clin Endocrinol Metab. 1993;77(1):216–20.
15. Giustina A, Veldhuis JD. Pathophysiology of the neuroregulation of growth hormone secretion in experimental animals and the human. Endocr Rev. 1998;19(6):717–97.
16. Gibney J, Healy ML, Sonksen PH. The growth hormone/insulin-like growth factor-I axis in exercise and sport. Endocr Rev. 2007;28(6):603–24.
17. Baxter RC. Insulin-like growth factor binding proteins in the human circulation: a review. Horm Res. 1994;42(4–5):140–4.
18. Jones JI, Clemmons DR. Insulin-like growth factors and their binding proteins: biological actions. Endocr Rev. 1995;16(1):3–34.
19. Ohlsson C, Bengtsson BA, Isaksson OG, Andreassen TT, Slootweg MC. Growth hormone and bone. Endocr Rev. 1998;19(1):55–79.
20. Seibel MJ. Molecular markers of bone turnover: biochemical, technical and analytical aspects. Osteoporos Int. 2000;11(Suppl 6):S18–29.
21. McHugh CM, Park RT, Sonksen PH, Holt RI. Challenges in detecting the abuse of growth hormone in sport. Clin Chem. 2005;51(9):1587–93.
22. Sonksen PH. Insulin, growth hormone and sport. J Endocrinol. 2001;170(1):13–25.
23. Wallace JD, Cuneo RC, Baxter R, et al. Responses of the growth hormone (GH) and insulin-like growth factor axis to exercise, GH administration, and GH withdrawal in trained adult males: a potential test for GH abuse in sport. J Clin Endocrinol Metab. 1999; 84(10):3591–601.
24. Wallace JD, Cuneo RC, Lundberg PA, et al. Responses of markers of bone and collagen turnover to exercise, growth hormone (GH) administration, and GH withdrawal in trained adult males. J Clin Endocrinol Metab. 2000;85(1):124–33.
25. Juul A. Serum levels of insulin-like growth factor I and its binding proteins in health and disease. Growth Horm IGF Res. 2003;13(4):113–70.
26. Szulc P, Seeman E, Delmas PD. Biochemical measurements of bone turnover in children and adolescents. Osteoporos Int. 2000;11(4):281–94.
27. Crofton PM, Wade JC, Taylor MR, Holland CV. Serum concentrations of carboxyl-terminal propeptide of type I procollagen, amino-terminal propeptide of type III procollagen, cross-linked carboxyl-terminal telopeptide of type I collagen, and their interrelationships in schoolchildren. Clin Chem. 1997;43(9):1577–81.
28. Healy ML, Dall R, Gibney J, et al. Toward the development of a test for growth hormone (GH) abuse: a study of extreme physiological ranges of GH-dependent markers in 813 elite athletes in the postcompetition setting. J Clin Endocrinol Metab. 2005;90(2):641–9.
29. Erotokritou-Mulligan I, Bassett EE, Cowan DA, et al. Influence of ethnicity on IGF-I and procollagen III peptide (P-III-P) in elite athletes and its effect on the ability to detect GH abuse. Clin Endocrinol (Oxf). 2009;70(1):161–8.
30. Nguyen TV, Nelson AE, Howe CJ, et al. Within-subject variability and analytic imprecision of insulin like growth factor axis and collagen markers: implications for clinical diagnosis and doping tests. Clin Chem. 2008;54(8):1268–76.
31. Holt RI, Erotokritou-Mulligan I, Ridley SA, et al. A determination of the pre-analytical storage conditions for insulin like growth factor-I and type III procollagen peptide. Growth Horm IGF Res. 2009;19(1):43–50.

32. Dall R, Longobardi S, Ehrnborg C, et al. The effect of four weeks of supraphysiological growth hormone administration on the insulin-like growth factor axis in women and men. GH-2000 Study Group. J Clin Endocrinol Metab. 2000;85(11):4193–200.
33. Longobardi S, Keay N, Ehrnborg C, et al. Growth hormone (GH) effects on bone and collagen turnover in healthy adults and its potential as a marker of GH abuse in sports: a double blind, placebo-controlled study. The GH-2000 Study Group. J Clin Endocrinol Metab. 2000;85(4): 1505–12.
34. Kniess A, Ziegler E, Kratzsch J, Thieme D, Muller RK. Potential parameters for the detection of hGH doping. Anal Bioanal Chem. 2003;376(5):696–700.
35. Sartorio A, Agosti F, Marazzi N, et al. Combined evaluation of resting IGF-I, N-terminal propeptide of type III procollagen (PIIINP) and C-terminal cross-linked telopeptide of type I collagen (ICTP) levels might be useful for detecting inappropriate GH administration in athletes: a preliminary report. Clin Endocrinol (Oxf). 2004;61(4):487–93.
36. Ehrnborg C, Ohlsson C, Mohan S, Bengtsson BA, Rosen T. Increased serum concentration of IGFBP-4 and IGFBP-5 in healthy adults during one month's treatment with supraphysiological doses of growth hormone. Growth Horm IGF Res. 2007;17(3):234–41.
37. Powrie JK, Bassett EE, Rosen T, et al. Detection of growth hormone abuse in sport. Growth Horm IGF Res. 2007;17(3):220–6.
38. Erotokritou-Mulligan I, Bassett EE, Kniess A, Sonksen PH, Holt RI. Validation of the growth hormone (GH)-dependent marker method of detecting GH abuse in sport through the use of independent data sets. Growth Horm IGF Res. 2007;17(5):416–23.
39. Nelson AE, Howe CJ, Nguyen TV, et al. Erythropoietin administration does not influence the GH--IGF axis or makers of bone turnover in recreational athletes. Clin Endocrinol (Oxf). 2005;63(3):305–9.
40. Kurdy NM, Bowles S, Marsh DR, Davies A, France M. Serology of collagen types I and III in normal healing of tibial shaft fractures. J Orthop Trauma. 1998;12(2):122–6.
41. Stoffel K, Engler H, Kuster M, Riesen W. Changes in biochemical markers after lower limb fractures. Clin Chem. 2007;53(1):131–4.
42. Erotokritou-Mulligan I, Bassett EE, Bartlett C, et al. The effect of sports injury on insulin-like growth factor-I and type 3 procollagen: implications for detection of growth hormone abuse in athletes. J Clin Endocrinol Metab. 2008;93(7):2760–3.
43. Bidlingmaier M, Strasburger CJ. Technology insight: detecting growth hormone abuse in athletes. Nat Clin Pract Endocrinol Metab. 2007;3(11):769–77.
44. Vignali DA. Multiplexed particle-based flow cytometric assays. J Immunol Methods. 2000; 243(1–2):243–55.
45. Kirsch S, Widart J, Louette J, Focant JF, De Pauw E. Development of an absolute quantification method targeting growth hormone biomarkers using liquid chromatography coupled to isotope dilution mass spectrometry. J Chromatogr A. 2007;1153(1–2):300–6.
46. Han B, Copeland M, Geiser AG, et al. Development of a highly sensitive, high-throughput, mass spectrometry-based assay for rat procollagen type-I N-terminal propeptide (PINP) to measure bone formation activity. J Proteome Res. 2007;6(11):4218–29.
47. Sharpe K, Ashenden MJ, Schumacher YO. A third generation approach to detect erythropoietin abuse in athletes. Haematologica. 2006;91(3):356–63.

Chapter 16
Distinction Between Endogenous and Exogenous Erythropoietin: Marker Methods

Jordi Segura and Mario Zorzoli

Erythropoietin (EPO) is a hormone synthesized predominantly in the kidneys that prevents the apoptosis [1] of red blood cell precursors in the bone marrow [2–5]. The increase in circulating erythrocytes can be used to increase delivery of oxygen to muscle, which improves performance in sport [6]. The availability of products of recombinant human EPO (rhEPO) has allowed its extended use. The authorities of sports forbade the use of EPO in 1988 and now any analog or mimetic is also included in the list of prohibited substances of the World Antidoping Agency (WADA). The challenge of detecting the misuse of EPO has given strength to the proposal of several strategies [7]. The physiological and biochemical effects of its administration can be used to suspect the application of the hormone. This is the basis of the so-called indirect or markers methods. They rely on the measurement of some hematologic and serum parameters and their comparison with populational or individual limit values. Recently, the latter approach has prompted the idea of the so-called Biological Passport, as a tool that will allow early identification of any hematological abnormality in specific parameters for a given subject indicative of a potential blood-doping activity. A reduced intermethodological and interlaboratory variability is of importance for the global application of such an approach [8]. This chapter is intended to gain insight into the indirect methodologies to detect the misuse of rhEPO in sport.

Models of Detection of Increased Erythropoiesis

The indirect methods require extraction of blood for the quantification of some parameters either in whole blood or in serum [9, 10]. Deep research has led to the proposal of mathematical models to detect an altered erythropoiesis. The use of

J. Segura (✉)

Bioanalysis Research Group, Neuropsychopharmacology Program, IMIM-Hospital del Mar, carrer Dr. Aiguader 88, 08003 Barcelona, Spain

e-mail: jsegura@imim.es

more than one parameter increases the sensitivity, reducing the possibilities of a false positive. Those multiparametric models are based on usual hematologic techniques and common clinical analyzers, although some models [11] include also the determination of the messenger RNA for some proteins by quantitative PCR. The first mathematical models included determination of hematocrit (Hct; portion of volume of whole blood occupied by erythrocytes), hematocrit of reticulocytes (retHct; portion of volume of whole blood occupied by reticulocytes), and percentage of macrocytic erythrocytes (%macro; percentage of erythrocytes with a cellular volume greater than 120 fL) in whole blood, as well as concentrations of EPO ([EPO]) and soluble receptors of transferrin ([sTfR]) in serum. The two initial models (ON: detection during the administration of EPO, and OFF: detection after having interrupted the administration of EPO) were the following [12, 13]:

$$ON = 3.721 \, Hct + 30.45 \, retHct + 0.1871 \ln [EPO] + 0.1267 \ln [sTfR]$$
$$+ 0.115 \ln [\%macro + 0.1]$$

$$OFF = 6.149 \, Hct - 92.87 \, retHct - 0.1463 \ln [EPO]$$

All the parameters implied in the previous equations except retHct were already known to be affected by changes in the erythropoiesis. A new parameter retHct was proposed to contribute to the detection of subjects with a change artificially induced in the rate of production of erythrocytes because it was known that the quantity of reticulocytes as well as its mean cellular volume were affected by the erythropoiesis. However, some disadvantages of those models were associated with the dependence from the cellular volume for some of the parameters, potentially affected by the storage of the blood and the conditions of transport. Another issue was the fact that some variables were not widely standardized in their measurement and could only be measured with certain types of analyzers. Therefore, a second generation of models with greater robustness and simpler application were suggested [14]. The new equations used concentrations of hemoglobin ([Hb]), EPO, and soluble receptors of transferrin as well as the percentage of reticulocytes (%ret; percentage of reticulocytes in comparison with the total quantity of erythrocytes; see [15] for the role of reticulocytes in sport medicine). Two sets of equations for every model ON and OFF were suggested. They were labeled additionally with the letters h, e, r, and s according to the parameters ([Hb], [EPO], %ret, and [sTfR], respectively) applied in every case, as follows:

$$ON\text{-}he = Hb + 9.74 \ln [EPO]; \quad ON\text{-}hes = Hb + 6.62 \ln [EPO] + 19.4 \ln [sTfR]$$

$$OFF\text{-}hr = Hb - 60 \, (\%ret)^{1/2}; \quad OFF\text{-}hre = Hb - 50 \, (\%ret)^{1/2} - 7 \ln [EPO]$$

The decision of using ON-he in front of ON-hes and OFF-hr in front of OFF-hre is a balance between availability of reagents, working costs, and the degree of efficiency of detection. When the tests were applied to different situations, the OFF models showed a better capacity of detection than the ON models . It is interesting to note that the ON and OFF parameters are not increased by other potentially

Table 16.1 ON and OFF parameters do not evolve toward false positive results by intermittent hypobaric exposure

| | Control | Hypobaric chamber | | Control | Hypobaric chamber | | |
| | | First day | | | Last day | | 14 Days after last day |
	First day	Pre-session	Post-session	Last day	Pre-session	Post-session	
Hb (g/L)	150	146	143	143	139	143	135
%ret (%)	0.8	0.8	0.9	1	0.7	0.7	0.8
EPO (IU/L)	10.7	8.3	16.6	10.8	4.6	24.8	9.2
ON-he	173.1	166.6	170.4	166.2	153.9	174.3	156.6
OFF-hr	96.3	92.3	86.1	83.0	88.8	92.8	81.3

Exposures to hypobaric chamber were 3 h/5 days/week for 4 weeks. Mean values corresponding to one reference (control) and one (hypobaric chamber) test group of eight trained triathlon athletes in each group. See [16] for other details

confusing hypoxic situations, which alter the endogenous EPO production, such as the hypobaric chamber intermittent hypoxia exposure (Table 16.1) used by some sportsmen.

On the other hand, the individual longitudinal follow-up could be more promising than the comparison with limit values of populational origin. As a result, the so-called third generation models will compare parameters obtained from a specific subject along time and estimate the probability that a multiparametric deviation might be caused by the administration of a doping product [17–19].

Newer approaches, such as the use of endogenous substances involved in the production of nitric oxide have also been mentioned as potential indirect markers of rhEPO administration. Specifically, dimethylarginine together with arginine and citruline have been preliminarily studied [20]. The rejuvenation of red blood cells after rhEPO administration may also be advantageously used by measurement of erythrocyte aspartate aminotransferase activity. An increased activity in subjects residents in low altitude could be indicative of rhEPO administration [21]. Alternatively, the reticulocyte maturation status, affected by rhEPO, could be studied by flow cytometric detection of transferrin receptor CD71 [22].

Genomic approaches to detect altered erythropoiesis will emerge also as indirect markers, using the rapidly evolving array methodologies, although their actual impact to improve the detection capability to indicate rhEPO abuse remains to be demonstrated. A preliminary work done with quantitative rtPCR already pointed toward mRNA for erythroid target genes, ferritin-light chain, and ornithine decarboxylase antizyme as potential markers [23].

An advantage of indirect methods to detect rhEPO is its universal coverage of different types of analogous and mimetics, a field in clear expansion. Thus, in 2001, and with the end of the protection of the patent of rhEPO in sight, Amgen introduced the darbepoetin alpha (NESP or ARANESP). More recently, Shire marketed Dynepo, a compound produced through the activation of the endogenous gene in a cell line of human fibrosarcoma.

Many other recombinant products, some of them of doubtful origin, have appeared or will appear soon in the market [24]. Additionally, synthetic analogs are already appearing as the synthetic erythropoiesis protein (SEP) [25] and the continuous activator of the erythropoiesis receptor (CERA) [26]. They all will give rise to changes in the indirect parameters similar to those of rhEPO described previously.

Analytical Variability of Some Biomarkers

Some factors distorting results when longitudinal studies are to be followed are the inherent known variability of clinical and immunological methods in general, the potential changes among reagent sets of antibodies, and the lack of harmonization for the standardization of the tests [27, 28]. Of highlighted interest for the indirect models mentioned above is the reliability of the measurements of hemoglobin and reticulocytes and also the immunological assays for EPO and for soluble receptors of transferrin in serum.

Hemoglobin values are influenced by genetic and environmental elements which lead to a large interindividual variability [29], while intraindividual variability can depend on many factors, especially plasma volume changes, which can be modified by interventions such as hydration, posture, altitude, or training. This is why [Hb] can change considerably in athletes and variations up to 10% are generally accepted [30, 31]. From the analytical point of view, Hb measurement has been standardized and its analytical variation is small.

On the contrary, reticulocytes measurement, which is more sensible in indentifying bone marrow changes due to blood doping, is a much more delicate parameter, especially in regard to analytical variability. In fact, if compared to hemoglobin, reticulocytes show a much larger analytical variability, due to a lack of calibration materials and different technologies integrated in automatic analyzers [15], which leads to important variations when applying different technologies. It is therefore necessary to decrease the analytical variability by applying one single technology or by correcting results obtained by different systems [28]. Additionally, reticulocytes are more easily influenced by external factors, not necessarily linked to blood doping, like storage temperature or the time delay between sampling and analysis. Therefore, standardized preanalytical and analytical procedures, which address all these issues, have to be implemented and respected.

Regarding measurements in serum, several comparisons of immunoassays for EPO have been published [13, 32–36]. A study addressed specifically to the analysis of EPO for the indirect models described here has been carried out [37], comparing an assay of chemiluminescence with an assay of ELISA, both of them previously used in the development of the mathematical models mentioned above. Similarly, there exist a great quantity of tests to determine soluble receptors of transferrin, the most predominant being the sandwich ELISA with monoclonal or polyclonal antibodies and measurements by turbidimetry or nephelometry. Again, several comparison studies have appeared [13, 38–46]. Appropriate equations must be applied when comparing results for soluble transferring receptors obtained by different techniques [47].

The outcome of studies in this field is that the exhaustive validation of the methods is of high importance for purposes of comparison, including intralaboratory, interlaboratory, and intertechnique variabilities.

Indirect Markers for Health Prevention: Health Tests

In addition to provide fair competition, one of the goals of the fight against doping is to protect athletes' health from the side effects of doping substances and methods, which could even lead to death in some cases (i.e., transfusional accident). The side effects of rhEPO are very well described in the literature [48], and of major concern are thromboembolic events, which could also be facilitated by the dehydration that occurs especially in endurance disciplines: those that are most influenced by the ergogenic effect of rhEPO. In the 1990s, there were rumors that rhEPO was used by athletes and that some of them put their life at risk while doing so, by increasing their Hct or Hb in an uncontrolled way to extremely high values (higher than 60% and 20 g/dL). They were encouraged in doing so by the rhEPO clear ergogenic effect due to the increase of the VO_2max [49], and by the fact that although prohibited by the International Olympic Committee since 1988, no antidoping test was available for its detection; therefore athletes were not at risk of being caught with traditional urine doping controls. Nevertheless, because administration of rhEPO induces a physiological response reflected in changes in easily measurable hematological parameters, different sporting authorities decided to introduce the so-called Hct or Hb rule. In fact, the idea was to set a population limit for these parameters, and athletes tested right before the competitions were allowed to compete only if their values lied below the established threshold. In the example of the International Cycling Union (UCI) health tests program, launched in March 1997, samples were collected on site of the competition, in the morning before the departure of the race, on an unannounced way. They were immediately analyzed and results were available within 1 h after blood collection, and athletes were notified of the decision about their "aptitude" or "inaptitude" to compete. The aims of this rule were first to protect athletes' health by limiting the magnitude of possible rhEPO manipulation and therefore the health risks linked to the induced polycythemic status, and secondly to protect the fairness of the competition by applying the available deterrent strategy in regard to rhEPO use. When the urinary rhEPO detection test became available in 2001 [50], an additional application of the evaluation of these results was their use as screening tests to target further antidoping controls [51]. But the introduction of the urinary test also lead to a change in the way some athletes administered blood doping (i.v. administration of microdoses of rhEPO more distant in time from the competitions, but also the reintroduction of blood transfusions). The program had therefore to adapt to this evolving situation, and new parameters were added (%ret, the OFF-hr score, or free plasma Hb).

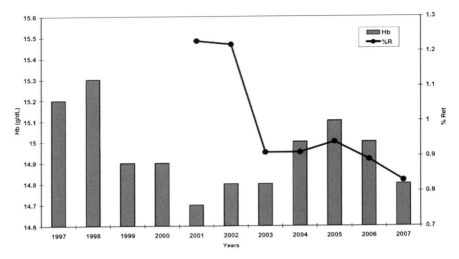

Fig. 16.1 Evolution of hemoglobin and reticulocytes. Mean [Hb] (*bars*) and %ret (*line*) in cyclists (mainly road male cyclists) from 1997 to 2007. Data are presented as means of each season. The left *y*-axis represents [Hb] and the right *y*-axis represents %ret. The *x*-axis represents seasons

Interestingly, the International Ski Federation (FIS) also confirmed, through the analysis of its results, this different use of blood doping. In fact, measuring those parameters, the same pattern was easily recognizable in both disciplines (cycling (Fig. 16.1) and cross-country skiing [19]): decrease of %ret, increase of Hb, and of OFF-hr score.

This was also reflected in the increased number of athletes declared inapt because of high OFF-hr score than for elevated Hct or Hb. It is the demonstration that the introduction of the OFF score has added more detection power in identifying athletes who might have used blood doping and found the way to lie within the established limits for Hct or Hb.

Indirect Markers for Doping Detection: Biological Passport

The increasing interest of the scientific community on indirect markers of doping detection (e.g. hematological parameters for blood doping or endocrinological parameters for growth hormone) has lead to the development of two different concepts: the individual longitudinal profile and the multivariable approach. When biological markers show an intra-athletes variability which is lower than inter-athletes variability, as it is the case with hematological parameters, individualized limits should be considered instead of applying the same cutoff for all [52, 53]. Already in 2003, Malcovati introduced the concept of an individual biological passport [31], where he proposed subject-specific reference ranges, which could be applied to distinguish between physiologic and abnormal variability as a consequence of diseases or blood doping. On the other hand, because each of these markers reacts differently to blood doping, and in order to increase their specificity and sensitivity, the combination of several parameters had been proposed. In 2006 and 2007, the WADA has gathered scientists and representatives of the sports federations involved in blood testing, in order to address the feasibility of the athlete's passport. It was agreed that, within the context of antidoping rules, some relevant hematological parameters should be monitored in and out of competition, and the athletes' results should be processed applying a Bayesian statistical approach [54, 55], which allows calculating the probability of abnormality of the profile. It was then agreed, that in order to decrease the variability due to the preanalytical and analytical factors, standardized protocols should be established and followed. These documents would address how blood samples should be collected, transported, and analyzed. Some major principles are: samples can be collected only 2 h after a physical effort (training or competition) [56]; only one sample can be collected; refrigerated transport has to be assured [57]; analysis should be realized within 36 h from the time of the collection [58]. Other important issues are dealt with, such as the fact that only one technology should be used to measure these parameters, in order to decrease the variability associated to reticulocytes measurement [15], that a common external quality control should be available to all accredited laboratories, and that all the laboratories should apply the same procedures when calibrating the machines and analyzing the samples. In 2008, UCI and WADA agreed to launch a pilot project in cycling, which included more than 800 athletes, which were tested several times through the year in and out of competition. This approach has lead to the creation of individual profiles which, after having been processed by the Abnormal Blood Profile software [59] (which applies the Bayesian statistical calculus), are transmitted to independent experts. Once evaluated, and if the evidence of blood doping is strong, recommendations to UCI and WADA can be made in order to open procedures against those athletes with highly abnormal profiles. In fact, the 2009 World Anti-Doping Code allows the possibility to sanction an athlete for doping based on an abnormal blood or urine profile. In the coming years, new parameters could be validated and introduced for the purpose of a more efficient global fight against doping, based on indirect evidences of doping: urinary steroid profiles [17, 60] or the indirect markers of human growth hormone abuse [61, 62].

Conclusions

Different attempts have been done to approach the detection of EPO misuse in sport. As many of them are based on independent principles, they can be used in an even cooperative way for a greater capacity of detection. The indirect or marker

methods based on abnormal variation of erythropoiesis and on other biochemical
parameters, in addition to prevent health risks during competition in athletes with
very high hematological markers, allow suspecting the administration of EPO,
analogs, or mimetics, with the possibility to select the suspicious subjects for
further tests that provide greater direct evidence. To select subjects through indirect
methods to be further targeted by direct approaches is also useful in order to tackle
the increasing pharmaceutical developments of designer drugs and synthetic
analogs and mimetics of rhEPO. With the introduction of the 2009 new World
Anti-Doping Code, there is another opportunity left to the antidoping authorities to
identify potential antidoping rules violation through abnormal profiles established
by means of longitudinal individual follow-up (athletes' passport).

Acknowledgement JS thanks background funding support from Generalitat de Catalunya
(Consell Català de l'Esport and Departament d'Innovació, Universitat i Empresa) and from
Spanish Ministerio de Educacion, Política Social y Deporte (Consejo Superior de Deportes).

References

1. Jelkmann W. Erythropoietin after a century of research: younger than ever. Eur J Haematol. 2007; 78: 183–205.
2. Faulds D, Sorkin EM. Epoetin (recombinant human erythropoietin). A review of its pharmacodynamic and pharmacokinetic properties and therapeutic potential in anaemia and the stimulation of erythropoiesis. Drugs. 1989; 38: 863–899.
3. Lappin TR, Rich IN. Erythropoietin – the first 90 years. Clin Lab Haematol. 1996; 18: 137–145.
4. Lacombe C, Mayeux P. Biology of erythropoietin. Haematologica. 1998; 83: 724–732.
5. Maiese K, Li F, Chong ZZ. New avenues of exploration for erythropoietin. JAMA. 2005; 293: 90–95.
6. Badia R, de la Torre R, Segura J. Erythropoietin: potential abuse in sport and possible methods for its detection. Biol Clin Hematol. 1992; 14: 177–184.
7. Pascual JA, Belalcazar V, de Bolos C, Gutierrez R, Llop E, Segura J. Recombinant erythropoietin and analogues: a challenge for doping control. Ther Drug Monit. 2004; 26: 175–179.
8. Peltre G, Thormann W. Evaluation report of the EPO blood tests. Independent internal Review to the World Antidoping Agency. 2003; 1–5.
9. Audran M, Gareau R, Matecki S, Durand F, Chenard C, Sicart MT, Marion B, Bressolle F. Effects of erythropoietin administration in training athletes and possible indirect detection in doping control. Med Sci Sports Exerc. 1999; 31: 639–645.
10. Breymann C. Erythropoietin test methods. Baillieres Best Pract Res Clin Endocrinol Metab. 2000; 14: 135–145.
11. Magnani M, Corsi D, Bianchi M, Paiardini M, Galluzzi L, Gargiullo E, Parisi A, Pigozzi F. Identification of blood erythroid markers useful in revealing erythropoietin abuse in athletes. Blood Cells Mol Dis. 2001; 27: 559–571.
12. Parisotto R, Gore CJ, Emslie KR, Ashenden MJ, Brugnara C, Howe C, Martin DT, Trout GJ, Hahn AG. A novel method utilising markers of altered erythropoiesis for the detection of recombinant human erythropoietin abuse in athletes. Haematologica. 2000; 85: 564–572.
13. Parisotto R, Wu M, Ashenden MJ, Emslie KR, Gore CJ, Howe C, Kazlauskas R, Sharpe K, Trout GJ, Xie M. Detection of recombinant human erythropoietin abuse in athletes utilizing markers of altered erythropoiesis. Haematologica. 2001; 86: 128–137.

14. Gore CJ, Parisotto R, Ashenden MJ, Stray-Gundersen J, Sharpe K, Hopkins W, Emslie KR, Howe C, Trout GJ, Kazlauskas R, Hahn AG. Second-generation blood tests to detect erythropoietin abuse by athletes. Haematologica. 2003; 88: 333–344.
15. Banfi G. Reticulocytes in sports medicine. Sports Med. 2008; 38: 187–211.
16. Abellan R, Ventura R, Remacha AF, Rodríguez FA, Pascual JA, Segura J. Intermittent hypoxia exposure in hypobaric chamber and EPO abuse Interpretation. J Sports Sci. 2007; 25: 1241–1250.
17. Robinson N, Sottas PE, Mangin P, Saugy M. Bayesian detection of abnormal hematological values to introduce a no-start rule for heterogeneous populations of athletes. Haematologica. 2007; 92: 1143–1144.
18. Sharpe K, Ashenden MJ, Schumacher YO. A third generation approach to detect erythropoietin abuse in athletes. Haematologica. 2006; 91: 356–363.
19. Morkeberg J, Saltin B, Belhage B, Damsgaard R. Blood profiles in elite cross-country skiers: a 6-year follow-up. Scand J Med Sci Sports. 2008; 19: 198–205.
20. Appolonova SA, Dikunets MA, Rodchenkov GM. Possible indirect detection of rHuEPO administration in human urine by high-performance liquid chromatography tandem mass spectrometry. Eur J Mass Spectrom (Chichester, Eng). 2008; 14: 201–209.
21. Robinson Y, Cristancho E, Boning D. Erythrocyte aspartate aminotransferase activity as a possible indirect marker for stimulated erythropoiesis in male and female athletes. Lab Hematol. 2007; 13: 49–55.
22. Borrione P, Parisi A, Salvo RA, Spaccamiglio A, Pautasso M, Baraban D, Piccoli GB, Pigozzi F, Angeli A. A peculiar pattern of expression of the transferrin receptor (CD71) by reticulocytes in patients given recombinant human erythropoietin (rHuEPO): a novel marker for abuse in sport? J Biol Regul Homeost Agents. 2007; 21: 79–88.
23. Varlet-Marie E, Audran M, Lejeune M, Bonafoux B, Sicart MT, Marti J, Piquemal D, Commes T. Analysis of human reticulocyte genes reveals altered erythropoiesis: potential use to detect recombinant human erythropoietin doping. Haematologica. 2004; 89: 991–997.
24. Macdougall IC, Ashenden M. Current and upcoming erythropoiesis-stimulating agents, iron products, and other novel anemia medications. Adv Chronic Kidney Dis. 2009; 16: 117–130.
25. Kochendoerfer GG, Chen SY, Mao F, Cressman S, Traviglia S, Shao H, Hunter CL, Low DW, Cagle EN, Carnevali M, Gueriguian V, Keogh PJ, Porter H, Stratton SM, Wiedeke MC, Wilken J, Tang J, Levy JJ, Miranda LP, Crnogorac MM, Kalbag S, Botti P, Schindler-Horvat J, Savatski L, Adamson JW, Kung A, Kent SB, Bradburne JA. Design and chemical synthesis of a homogeneous polymer-modified erythropoiesis protein. Science. 2003; 299: 884–887.
26. Macdougall IC. CERA (Continuous Erythropoietin Receptor Activator): a new erythropoiesis-stimulating agent for the treatment of anemia. Curr Hematol Rep. 2005; 4: 436–440.
27. Lippi G, Guidi G. Laboratory screening for erythropoietin abuse in sport: an emerging challenge. Clin Chem Lab Med. 2000; 38: 13–19.
28. Ashenden MJ, Sharpe K, Damsgaard R, Jarvis L. Standardization of reticulocyte values in an antidoping context. Am J Clin Pathol. 2004; 121: 816–825.
29. Sala C, Ciullo M, Lanzara C, Nutile T, Bione S, Massacane R, d'Adamo P, Gasparini P, Toniolo D, Camaschella C. Variation of hemoglobin levels in normal Italian populations from genetic isolates. Haematologica. 2008; 93: 1372–1375.
30. Engelmeyer E, deMarées M, Achtzehn S, Lundby C, Saltin B, Mester J. Inter- and intra-individual variations of Hb concentration with different interventions in elite cross country skiers. 12th Annual Congress of ECSS. 2007.
31. Malcovati L, Pascutto C, Cazzola M. Hematologic passport for athletes competing in endurance sports: a feasibility study. Haematologica. 2003; 88: 570–581.
32. Bechensteen AG, Lappin TR, Marsden J, Muggleston D, Cotes PM. Unreliability in immunoassays of erythropoietin: anomalous estimates with an assay kit. Br J Haematol. 1993; 83: 663–664.

33. Lindstedt G, Lundberg PA. Are current methods of measurement of erythropoietin (EPO) in human plasma or serum adequate for the diagnosis of polycythaemia vera and the assessment of EPO deficiency? Scand J Clin Lab Invest. 1998; 58: 441–458.
34. Marsden JT, Sherwood RA, Peters TJ. Evaluation of six erythropoietin kits. Ann Clin Biochem. 1999; 36 (Pt 3): 380–387.
35. Benson EW, Hardy R, Chaffin C, Robinson CA, Konrad RJ. New automated chemiluminescent assay for erythropoietin. J Clin Lab Anal. 2000; 14: 271–273.
36. Owen WE, Roberts WL. Performance characteristics of the IMMUNLITE 2000 erythropoietin assay. Clin Chim Acta. 2004; 340: 213–217.
37. Abellan R, Ventura R, Pichini S, Remacha AF, Pascual JA, Pacifici R, Di Giovannandrea R, Zuccaro P, Segura J. Evaluation of immunoassays for the measurement of erythropoietin (EPO) as an indirect biomarker of recombinant human EPO misuse in sport. J Pharm Biomed Anal. 2004; 35: 1169–1177.
38. Kuiper-Kramer EP, Huisman CM, van Raan J, van Eijk HG. Analytical and clinical implications of soluble transferrin receptors in serum. Eur J Clin Chem Clin Biochem. 1996; 34: 645–649.
39. Suominen P, Punnonen K, Rajamaki A, Irjala K. Evaluation of new immunoenzymometric assay for measuring soluble transferrin receptor to detect iron deficiency in anemic patients. Clin Chem. 1997; 43: 1641–1646.
40. Yeung GS, Kjarsgaard JC, Zlotkin SH. Disparity of serum transferrin receptor measurements among different assay methods. Eur J Clin Nutr. 1998; 52: 801–804.
41. Akesson A, Bjellerup P, Vahter M. Evaluation of kits for measurement of the soluble transferrin receptor. Scand J Clin Lab Invest. 1999; 59: 77–81.
42. Suominen P, Punnonen K, Rajamaki A, Majuri R, Hanninen V, Irjala K. Automated immunoturbidimetric method for measuring serum transferrin receptor. Clin Chem. 1999; 45: 1302–1305.
43. Cotton F, Thiry P, Boeynaems J. Measurement of soluble transferrin receptor by immunoturbidimetry and immunonephelometry. Clin Biochem. 2000; 33: 263–267.
44. Wians FH, Jr., Urban JE, Kroft SH, Keffer JH. Soluble transferrin receptor (sTfR) concentration quantified using two sTfR kits: analytical and clinical performance characteristics. Clin Chim Acta. 2001; 303: 75–81.
45. Paritpokee N, Bhokaisawan N, Wiwanitkit V, Boonchalermvichian C. Methodology evaluation of a new immunoturbidimetric method for measuring serum soluble transferrin receptor. Asian Pac J Allergy Immunol. 2001; 19: 207–211.
46. Thomas C, Thomas L. Biochemical markers and hematologic indices in the diagnosis of functional iron deficiency. Clin Chem. 2002; 48: 1066–1076.
47. Abellan R, Ventura R, Pichini S, Sarda MP, Remacha AF, Pascual JA, Palmi I, Bacosi A, Pacifici R, Zuccaro P, Segura J. Evaluation of immunoassays for the measurement of soluble transferrin receptor as an indirect biomarker of recombinant human erythropoietin misuse in sport. J Immunol Methods. 2004; 295: 89–99.
48. Lippi G, Franchini M, Salvagno GL, Guidi GC. Biochemistry, physiology, and complications of blood doping: facts and speculation. Crit Rev Clin Lab Sci. 2006; 43: 349–391.
49. Berglund B, Ekblom B. Effect of recombinant human erythropoietin treatment on blood pressure and some haematological parameters in healthy men. J Intern Med. 1991; 229: 125–130.
50. Lasne F, de Ceaurriz J. Recombinant erythropoietin in urine. Nature. 2000; 405: 635.
51. Zorzoli M. Recent advances in anti-doping settings. In: W. Schanzer, H. Geyer, A. Gotzmann, U. Marcck (eds) Recent advances in doping analysis (13). Sport und Buch Strauss, Köln. 2005; 255–264.
52. Harris EK. Effects of intra- and interindividual variation on the appropriate use of normal ranges. Clin Chem. 1974; 20: 1535–1542.
53. Ceriotti F, Hinzmann R, Panteghini M. Reference intervals: the way forward. Ann Clin Biochem. 2009; 46: 8–17.

54. Sottas PE, Robinson NE, Giraud S, Taroni F, Kamber M, Mangin P, Saugy M. Statistical classification of abnormal blood profiles in athletes. Int J Biostatistics. 2006; 2: 3.
55. Sottas PE, Robinson NE, Saugy M, Niggli O. A forensic approach to the interpretation of blood doping markers. Law Probability and Risk. 2008; 7: 191–210.
56. WADA. Athlete's Hematological Passport Blood Collection Protocol (to be released). www.wada-ama.org 2009.
57. WADA. Athlete's Hematological Passport Blood Storage and Transport Protocol (to be released). www.wada-ama.org 2009.
58. WADA. Athlete's Hematological Passport Blood Analytical Protocol (to be released). www.wada-ama.org 2009.
59. WADA. Athlete's Hematological Passport Interpretation Technical Document (to be released). www.wada-ama.org 2009.
60. Sottas PE, Saudan C, Schweizer C, Baume N, Mangin P, Saugy M. From population- to subject-based limits of T/E ratio to detect testosterone abuse in elite sports. Forensic Sci Int. 2008; 174: 166–172.
61. Powrie JK, Bassett EE, Rosen T, Jorgensen JO, Napoli R, Sacca L, Christiansen JS, Bengtsson BA, Sonksen PH. Detection of growth hormone abuse in sport. Growth Horm IGF Res. 2007; 17: 220–226.
62. Erotokritou-Mulligan I, Bassett EE, Kniess A, Sonksen PH, Holt RI. Validation of the growth hormone (GH)-dependent marker method of detecting GH abuse in sport through the use of independent data sets. Growth Horm IGF Res. 2007; 17: 416–423.

Chapter 17
Direct Methods for Distinction Between Endogenous and Exogenous Erythropoietin

Séverine Lamon, Neil Robinson, and Martial Saugy

Since the commercialization of the first recombinant human erythropoietin (rhEPO) product (epoetin-α) in 1989 as a treatment for acute anemia, rhEPO detection has represented a continuous challenge for the anti-doping fight. Indeed, it appeared rapidly that this ergogenic hormone would be abused by athletes looking for an artificial performance enhancer. Hemoglobin is one of the principal modulators of aerobic power [1, 2] and, consequently, of performance in endurance sports [3]. By stimulating the red blood cells production, EPO is known to raise hemoglobin concentration in a dose-dependant and predictable way. Therefore, this hormone soon became one of the athletes most popular doping agent. Since 1984, all forms of blood doping in sport have been officially banned. In 1990, the IOC medical commission, which was in charge of the anti-doping regulations, added rhEPO to the list of the prohibited drugs in sports, even if a direct test allowing to detect the molecule became available a decade after only.

History of rhEPO Direct Detection

The most powerful way to discriminate between endogenous and rhEPO is probably based on the glycosylation differences existing between both types of molecules. Indeed, glycosylation of rhEPO takes place in CHO cells rather than in human cells [4]. As a result, recombinant molecules exhibit fewer sialic acid residues on their surface. Hence, recombinant isoforms are less negatively charged than endogenous ones and this charge difference allows to distinguish between endogenous and exogenous EPO molecules [5].

In 1995, Wide et al. proposed for the first time a method able to separate both types of molecules in blood and urine [6]. The median charge of EPO was determined,

M. Saugy (✉)
Laboratoire Suisse d'Analyse du Dopage, Centre Universitaire Romand de Médecine Légale,
Centre Hospitalier Universitaire Vaudois and University of Lausanne, Epalinges, Switzerland
e-mail: martial.saugy@chuv.ch

E. Ghigo et al. (eds.), *Hormone Use and Abuse by Athletes*, Endocrine Updates 29,
DOI 10.1007/978-1-4419-7014-5_17, © Springer Science+Business Media, LLC 2011

either in blood or in urine concentrates, thanks to an electrophoresis in a 0.1% agarose suspension and was then expressed in terms of electrophoretic mobility. This technique was reliable, as it allowed to clearly identify the presence of rhEPO in urine and blood. However, while the proposed method was powerful as long as the biological samples were collected within 24 h after the last rhEPO injection, it appeared to be far less sensitive on samples having been collected later after injection. Indeed, after 3 days following the last rhEPO injection, no rhEPO traces could be found in more than half of the subjects. Furthermore, no sample presented any trace of rhEPO after 7 days following the last injection. Nevertheless, this study showed for the first time that administered rhEPO could be directly detected in urine. In contrast to the indirect rhEPO abuse detection models, this method had the undeniable advantage to attest the presence of the drug itself in biological fluids. It appeared, however, to be time-consuming and expensive. Moreover, it could not be settled in another laboratory and, therefore, was never applied in the anti-doping context.

The Isoelectric Focusing Test

In June 2000 – a few weeks before the Sydney Olympic games – Lasne and De Ceaurriz [7] presented an innovative test based on the isoelectric separation of urinary EPO isoforms on a polyacrylamide gel followed by a double blotting process [8, 9]. The principle of this method was still based on the charge differences existing between the endogenous and the recombinant hormone. Indeed, isoelectric focusing (IEF) allows the separation of proteins regarding their individual isoelectric points. The isoforms of epoetin-α and -β, both representatives of the first generation of recombinant EPOs, were demonstrated to be less acidic than the endogenous isoforms of human EPO (hEPO) [10] (Fig. 17.1). Thus, a particular isoelectric pattern could be defined for each EPO form [11]. In spite of the fact that IEF was as expensive and time-consuming as the method proposed by Wide, it appeared to be reproducible and reliable and therefore, worthwhile in the anti-doping context. Breidbach et al. rapidly assessed the sensitivity of the method [12]. In 2003, they observed that all the subjects having received nine injections of 50 IU/kg epoetin-α were detectable 3 days after the last EPO injection. Moreover, on the seventh day after the last rhEPO dose, approximately half of the subjects still showed rhEPO traces in their urine. In spite of difficult beginnings, notably due to the ineffective strategy adopted to fight against rhEPO doping during the Sydney Olympic games, IEF finally impose itself as the official test recommended by the World Anti-Doping Agency (WADA) for the detection of rhEPO abuse in athletes. In 2001, the laboratory of Lausanne reported the first positive rhEPO doping case that incriminated the Danish cyclist Bo Hamburger. This case was brought in front of the court (Court of Arbitration for Sport [CAS], Lausanne). At that time, discrepancies existed between the laboratories of Lausanne and Paris concerning the criteria that had to be fulfilled to declare a case positive. Indeed, Lausanne requested that 80% of the EPO bands had to be located in the basic area of the gel, while Paris set this limit at 85%. This incoherency caused

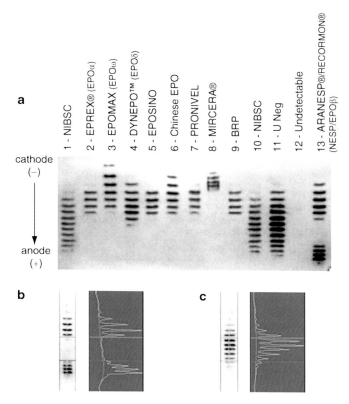

Fig. 17.1 (**a**) IEF gel with usual positive controls (ARANESP®/RECORMON®) standards, lane 13, Biological Reference Preparation (BRP) standard, lane 9, and negative control (NIBSC [National Institute for Biological Standards and Control] standard, lanes 1 and 10). Note that ARANESP® is a second generation EPO (NESP). Lanes 2–7 represent first generation EPOs, including copy EPOs (lanes 5–7). Lane 8 represents a third generation EPO (CERA). Lane 11 represents a negative urine. Lane 12 depicts an undetectable pattern. (**b**) Integration of ARANESP® and RECORMON® standards. A "basic area" is defined from the cathode edge up to and including band 1 of BRP, while an "acid area" is defined from the anode edge up to and including band A of ARANESP®. Relative intensities are then attributed to each defined band. (**c**) Integration of a negative urine pattern

the lost of the case. However, a few years later, Hamburger openly admitted to have abused of rhEPO. Nowadays, the positivity criteria are harmonized and stated in the WADA EPO technical document [13], which is regularly updated.

Initially, the test was designed to separate the classical first generation EPOs (epoetin-α, -β, and -ω) from hEPO in urine. During the nine last years, it has been adapted to other recombinant EPO forms, like darbepoetin-α (NESP, novel erythropoiesis-stimulating protein, second generation EPO), whose isoforms are located in the most acidic part of the gel, epoetin-δ (DYNEPO™) or, more recently, generic (biosimilar) or "copy" EPOs. The rapid and incessant evolution of the anti-doping problem continually triggers the test development. Among other actual evolutions, the sample preparation technique, which is basically constituted of several concentration and ultrafiltration steps allowing to concentrate 20 ml of urine to 20–40 µl of an urinary extract called retentate, shall undergo significant changes. The improvement of the quality and the purity of EPO extracts, as well as the extraction of EPO from the blood matrix, constitute the main actual challenges. Immunoaffinity-based techniques, like the ones recently proposed by Lasne [14] or Lönnberg [15], probably constitute the most promising tool to reach this goal. One of the main advantage of combining immunoaffinity and IEF resides is the use of two distinct anti-EPO antibodies in the same procedure, which is of major importance to exclude all types of cross-reactions with unspecific antigens. Indeed, it is important to mention that, despite the fact that IEF is currently the only official, accredited EPO screening method used on a routine basis in the anti-doping laboratories, numerous controversial articles have been published since 2000, disputing one or other aspect of the method. In 2006, Franke challenged scientific parameters of the IEF and aimed at proving that it was not suitable for anti-doping purposes [16]. Principally, and like other authors [17–19], he questioned the specificity of the anti-EPO antibody – the AE7A5 clone, a monoclonal mouse antibody manufactured by R&D systems – recommended by WADA for IEF. Proposing a new two-dimensional (2D) gel-based separation method, Khan et al. notably claimed the existence of several urinary proteins cross-reacting with the AE7A5 clone and suggested that false-positive results may have been returned [19]. IEF experts responded by mentioning the very poor quality of the presented 2D gels as well as the total absence of any bands in the window used for interpretation of the isoelectric profiles in the case of samples devoid of EPO deposited on an IEF gel [20]. Nevertheless, in 2008, Reichel proved the existence of a nonspecifically interacting urinary protein identified as zinc-alpha-2-glycoprotein using a shotgun proteomics approach including nano-HPLC peptide separation and high-resolution high-mass accuracy ESI-MS/MS peptide sequencing [21]. However, it was also clearly shown that this binding occurred outside the used pH range for evaluating EPO profiles.

Atypical EPO Patterns

IEF occupies a particular place among classical anti-doping methods. Indeed, this purely biochemical method contrasts with the complex analytical tools used for the detection of most doping substances. Associated with the technique, new difficulties appeared. Among others, several particular cases referred to as "atypical patterns" can be a source of troubles in IEF results interpretation. Undetectable, effort and active urines are the most common of these patterns.

Undetectability of EPO in urine samples is a phenomenon that was reported shortly after the implementation of IEF as the official EPO screening test in the anti-doping laboratories. Indeed, in 2003, two external experts were mandated by WADA to produce an exhaustive report on the urine EPO test [22]. One of the improvements they proposed concerned the preconcentration step; indeed, following the 700- to 1,000-fold concentration resulting from the retentate preparation, quite a large number of samples did not show a measurable EPO profile. Basically, an EPO profile is considered as undetectable if no endogenous or recombinant EPO can be detected in the sample using the classical IEF-based test (see Fig. 17.1). At that time, six anti-doping laboratories were performing the EPO test. One of them even reported an undetectability percentage of more than 20% among routine samples. It was also stated that samples being unusually rich in proteins, especially those collected after an important physical effort, could induce some artifacts in the method. Defaults in electrophoretic migration inducing smears and excessive background staining were notably mentioned. In 2006, the LAD conducted a study that aimed at determining the possible origins of undetectable EPO profiles in athletes' urine [23]. Statistical analyses performed on 3,050 negative EPO routine samples indicated that undetectable EPO profiles were clearly related to urine properties such as low EPO concentrations or extremely low or high specific gravities. The possible usage of proteasic adulterants to evade doping detection was also considered. Indeed, the addition of very small quantities of protease was shown to remove all traces of EPOs in urine. This finding led to the development of a simple test revealing proteasic activity on the basis of albumin degradation.

Strenuous efforts also generate atypical patterns [18]. Since IEF was introduced on a routine basis, atypical, basic profiles have been punctually observed by the anti-doping laboratories (Fig. 17.2). At the beginning of the method, these atypical profiles, had not been described and therefore were not taken into account by the effective positivity criteria. Interestingly, these atypical patterns are known to be characteristic of urine

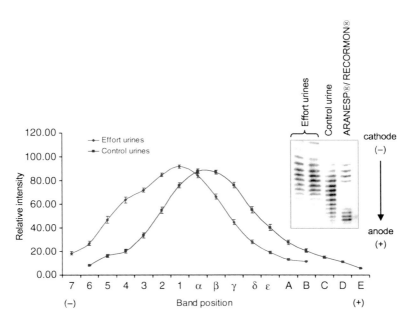

Fig. 17.2   Band distribution of control urines ($n=67$) and effort urines ($n=68$). As depicted on the gel, effort urines present a characteristic shift toward the basic area of the gel when compared with control urines. Error bars represent standard error of the mean (SEM)

samples collected after strenuous exercises. They are therefore commonly referred to as "effort urines." As a result, the WADA positivity criteria have been immediately adapted to take into account such atypical natural patterns in IEF interpretation: indeed, the former 80% rule that was previously followed to demonstrate the presence of rhEPO in urine was abolished. A strict position and distribution of the basic isoforms of the hormone, in terms of band position and intensity, had now to be respected. We recently showed that effort urines could be generated under precise controlled conditions and that supra-maximal short duration exercises induced the transformation of typical urinary natural EPO patterns into atypical ones. An exercise-induced transient renal dysfunction was proposed as a hypothetic explanation for these observations, which relies on parallel investigations of proteinuria in the same samples. Urinary retinol-binding protein (RBP) was proposed as a protein marker to identify effort urine samples (Fig. 17.3).

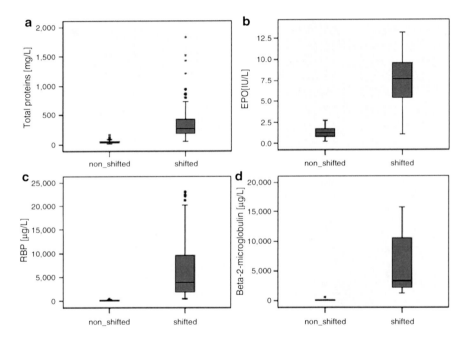

Fig. 17.3 Atypical urines due to strenuous efforts present significant differences when compared with normal, nonshifted urines. Total protein and EPO concentrations were notably shown to increase strikingly in effort urines. Ideally, a reliable protein marker that would be able to differentiate unequivocally between effort and normal urines should be determined. Beta-2-microglobulin was first suggested to play this role. It was recently proposed to rather use retinol-binding protein (RBP) concentrations as such a marker. Indeed, this small protein is a well-described indicator of tubular proteinuria, which was suggested to be part of the transient renal dysfunction that we proposed as an hypothesis for effort urines. (**a**) Total protein concentration (mg/l) in shifted ($n=93$) and nonshifted urines ($n=67$). (**b**) EPO concentration (IU/l) in shifted ($n=27$) and nonshifted urines ($n=67$). (**c**) RBP concentration (μg/ml) in shifted ($n=93$) and nonshifted urines ($n=67$). (**d**) Beta-2-microglobulin concentration (μg/ml) in shifted ($n=75$) and nonshifted urines ($n=23$)

Following the Lagat affair in 2003, a new parameter was considered to avoid the occurrence of false-positive cases; indeed, although Lagat's B-sample was tested negative, his A-sample presented an atypical, extremely basic EPO profile that was suggested to be due to a bacterial degradation of the urine. The conservation and transport conditions of the samples were therefore questioned. As a result, an additional assay, called stability test, was added to the WADA requirements for rhEPO screening. Stability test aims at demonstrating that no bacterial activity occurred in the urine. To this purpose, rhEPO and NESP are added to the sample before one night incubation at 37°C. The sample is then deposited on a gel and, in the case of the bands position of both EPO forms is not altered when compared with the corresponding controls, any bacterial activity can be excluded. Nowadays, no positive result can be returned without having performed a stability test.

First Generation EPO Generics: Biosimilars EPO

As recently reviewed by Macdougall and Ashenden [24], the emergence of biosimilars EPOs constitutes an extremely large investigation field for the fight against EPO abuse and shall strongly influence it in the future. Indeed, the patent for epoetin molecules expired in Europe in 2004. From then on, manufacturers have started to bring generics of epoetins, the so-called "biosimilars," on the market. At the time of writing, two such biosimilar epoetins have been approved by the EU and others may follow. However, a large number of "copy" recombinant EPOs are believed to be available worldwide. Copy EPOs are probably synthesized using similar techniques to the original products, even if their production process is usually not stringent and controlled enough to be approved by drug regulatory authorities such as the Food and Drug Administration in the United States and the European Medicines Agency in Europe. It was estimated that up to 80 such products may be sold in emergent countries. The appearance of biosimilar and copy EPOs represents a challenge for the fight against EPO doping. Indeed, due to the various production processes, slight differences can exist between the various EPO forms. Notably, the positions and intensities of isoforms can be somewhat modified. For example, Chinese EPO was shown to present a slightly more basic EPO pattern than epoetin-α and -β, but this small difference is sufficient to fail the pattern to fulfill all the three effective WADA positivity criteria, that take into account first and second generation EPO forms only (Fig. 17.1). Epoetin-δ (DYNEPO™) is a more recently engineered recombinant EPO that is produced by gene activation in human fibrosarcoma cells into which a DNA fragment, that activates the EPO promoter, was transfected [25]. Its isoforms are more alike the ones of endogenous EPO than other rhEPO, thus making things easier for cheating athletes. Therefore, the entire WADA politics toward these criteria may be rethought, as it is necessary to adapt them to the numerous EPO forms available on the market, considering their diversity in terms of bands position and distribution on the gel.

Second Generation EPO: NESP

NESP (darbepoetin-α), the first retard EPO product, was launched on the market by Amgen in June 2001 (ARANESP®). This second generation erythropoiesis-stimulating agent (ESA) has a prolonged survival in the blood circulation and therefore, aims at reducing the frequency of EPO injections in patients suffering from chronic kidney disease or other chronic disorders. As rhEPO, NESP derives from CHO cells. Both molecules can however be discriminated on an IEF gel thanks to glycosylation and primary structure differences. Soon after NESP approbation for medical use, its isoelectric pattern was observed in the urines of three athletes competing in the 2002 Winter Olympic Games in Salt Lake City. In 2005, a pilot excretion study of ARANESP® in human individuals was conducted, which aimed at determining its detection window after a single subcutaneous injection using the official IEF method [26]. Following a single 4,760 IU NESP injection, a detection window of a minimum of 7 days was observed, according to the WADA positivity criteria. This detection window was considerably longer than for rhEPO and therefore, NESP appeared to be probably a less adapted doping agent than rhEPO.

Third Generation EPO: CERA

CERA, a continuous erythropoietin receptor activator, is the active ingredient of a new drug for anemia treatment (MIRCERA®) developed by Roche. This first third-generation ESA is synthesized by the integration of a single large polyethylene glycol (PEG) chain into the epoetin molecule, thus increasing the molecular weight to twice that of epoetin [27]. It has been reported that the integration of PEG molecules may maintain in vivo biologic activity of some pharmaceutically active molecules [28]. For CERA, integration of the PEG moiety has resulted in an increased half-life and increased biologic activity in vivo when compared with epoetin. Patients treated with short-acting and frequently administered ESAs can be switched directly to once-monthly CERA without compromise in efficacy or safety [29]. To avoid illegal abuse of this new agent in sport, an enzyme-linked immuno-sorbent assay (ELISA) for the detection of CERA in blood was recently validated in collaboration with Roche. In a pilot clinical trial including six healthy subjects, the detection window of CERA in blood samples using the new method varied greatly among individuals, ranging between 8 and more than 27 days after a single 200 μg CERA administration. This long detection window suggests that CERA may not be the most convenient doping agent for sports performance, despite its major clinical advantage of increased dosing intervals. Nevertheless, the first CERA doping cases were recently reported. Indeed, during the Tour de France 2008, the Agence Française de Lutte contre le Dopage (AFLD) collected blood samples for anti-doping purposes and noticed suspicious hemograms. A total of 35 such samples were targeted and subjected to the ELISA test, yielding 27 values that were significantly smaller and 8 values that were significantly higher than the proposed threshold (Fig. 17.4). The presence of CERA could be confirmed in all the suspect samples

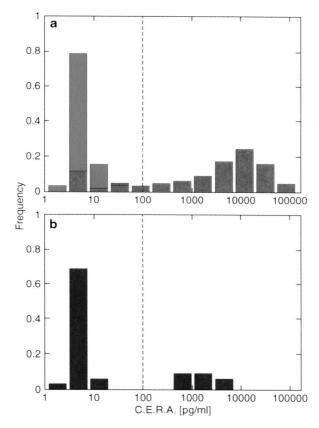

Fig. 17.4 (**a**) Histograms of CERA blood concentrations (pg/ml) in a population of control samples (*n* = 140 neat serum samples, one sample per subject, *green*) and in a population of positive samples (*n* = 56, *red*). Positive samples were collected in a pilot clinical trial involving six male healthy subjects having received 200 µg of CERA intravenously (three subjects) or subcutaneously (three subjects). All six subjects were followed over a period of 4 weeks. (**b**) Histogram of CERA blood concentrations (pg/ml) in a population of targeted athletes taking part to the Tour de France 2008 (*n* = 35, *blue*). Cut-off limit for the ELISA test was fixed at 100 pg/ml (*dashed line*)

using a variant of the classical IEF test adapted to the blood matrix. Thanks to its observed high discrimination power, the ELISA may therefore provide a valuable, complementary alternative to the IEF method in blood EPO testing.

Perspectives and Alternatives to the IEF Test

Since the publication of the IEF test in 2000, it has been subject to some controversies. These incessant challenges present, however, the advantage that the method has been incessantly questioned and that several groups have worked simultaneously at improving its sensitivity and specificity. New EPOs with variable

IEF profiles as well as active urines and effort urines have made additional strategies necessary. Active defenders of IEF recently revealed that the test still allowed athletes using rhEPO microdoses to evade doping controls [30], thus highlighting the necessity to continuously update the method and the corresponding positivity criteria. Alternative methods were also developed. In 2003, it was suggested that epoetin-α, -β, and NESP could be separated by means of 2D electrophoresis [31]. The main advantage of 2D-based methods resides in the separation of molecules by both their isoelectric point and molecular mass. However, the sensitivity of the proposed technique was far lower to consider its application for anti-doping purposes. Two years later, the group of Khan described a more sensitive 2D gel electrophoresis method [19] and suggested to definitely replace IEF by 2D. The technique was however subject to serious controversials [20].

During the last 10 years, the research of an IEF-orthogonal method, which could be used either as a screening or as a confirmation method, has occupied many scientists of the anti-doping field. Some of them developed the idea that hEPO and rhEPO molecules have a slightly different apparent molecular mass and proposed therefore a SDS-PAGE variant as a complementary method to IEF [32, 33]. Endogenous and exogenous EPOs are discriminated in term of relative electrophoretic mobility on a denaturant gel, the molecular masses of recombinant EPOs being typically higher than that of hEPO. While epoetins-α and -β showed rather subtle differences in electrophoretic mobility when compared with hEPO, this method appeared to be very beneficial in relation to active and effort urines. Moreover, epoetin-δ (DYNEPO™) presented a characteristic and clearly identifiable pattern, like darbepoeitin-α (NESP) or CERA. However, this may apparently not be the case for several copy EPOs that cannot be differentiated from hEPO using this method.

One of the most promising approaches for rhEPO screening in urine is certainly the membrane-assisted isoform immunoassay (MAIIA). This new technology recently developed by a Swedish group is able to distinguish minor differences in protein carbohydrate structure, requiring a very few amount of each isoform. MAIIA chips are micro-immunoaffinity columns composed of a separation zone, containing either anion exchange groups or ligands like lectins, and a capturing zone with immobilized specific antibodies. In the case of EPO isoforms detection, the separation zone contains wheat germ agglutinin groups, where isoforms interacting with the ligands are retarded. After having passed the separation zone, the weak binding isoforms are captured and detected in the antibody zone. This completely innovative technology is currently still being developed. Nevertheless, it may represent a powerful alternative to IEF in a few years.

Currently, complex analytical approaches based on mass spectrometry (MS) tools constitute the technique of choice for the screening of a large number of drugs in urine. As MS has demonstrated its utility for peptide and proteins on various occasions in the past, no conclusive approach has been however established for EPO. In 2005, epoetin-α, -β, and NESP could be differentiated by matrix-assisted laser desorption/ionization mass spectrometry (MALDI-MS) applying a high-resolution time-of-flight (TOF). The discrimination of the three molecules was based on the identification of distinct molecular substructures at the protein level triggered by specific enzymatic reactions [34]. In 2008, a method allowing the differentiation and identification of rhEPO and NESP in equine plasma by liquid-chromatography coupled to tandem mass spectrometry (LC-MS/MS) was published [35]. Recently, the same group proposed an extension of the proposed method in human plasma [36]. However, as this method is certainly powerful for the identification of NESP in human plasma, it is not applicable to rhEPO because it cannot differentiate the recombinant from the endogenous molecule. In addition, the extensive characterization that was achieved for rhEPO was never performed on human endogenous EPO because its standard is not available in sufficient amount [37]. The main encountered obstacles are probably the lack of sensitivity consequent of the very low amounts of EPO available in urine specimens, as well as the heterogeneity of endogenously produced and recombinant EPO molecules.

Conclusion

As WADA was founded, in 1999, one of the aims of the new agency was the harmonization of the results' interpretation in all anti-doping laboratories of the world. In the case of rhEPO, it led to the creation of a common technical document [13], and this certainly avoided the laboratories to repeat some errors of the past. The new organization also promoted the links between anti-doping laboratories and pharmaceutical industries. As illustrated by the CERA example, a close collaboration between both entities before a drug is put on the market represents an encouraging trend in the anti-doping field and shall allow, in the future, the emergence of rapid responses to new doping behaviors. In any cases, the fight against EPO doping must continue to adapt to the main actual trends such as the choice of rapid and simple screening tests associated to heavier confirmation assays, the always more common use of blood matrix or the secondary markers philosophy (biological passport) which, through an efficient athletes targeting, can strongly improve the efficiency of direct rhEPO detection. Indeed, reactivity is certainly a key element that contributes to foster the anti-doping fight, in general.

References

1. Kanstrup IL, Ekblom B. Blood volume and hemoglobin concentration as determinants of maximal aerobic power. Med Sci Sports Exerc. 1984;16(3):256–262.
2. Gledhill N, Warburton D, Jamnik V. Haemoglobin, blood volume, cardiac function, and aerobic power. Can J Appl Physiol. 1999;24(1):54–65.
3. Craig NP, Norton KI, Bourdon PC, et al. Aerobic and anaerobic indices contributing to track endurance cycling performance. Eur J Appl Physiol Occup Physiol. 1993;67(2):150–158.
4. Wang MD, Yang M, Huzel N, Butler M. Erythropoietin production from CHO cells grown by continuous culture in a fluidized-bed bioreactor. Biotechnol Bioeng. 2002;77(2):194–203.
5. Choi D, Kim M, Park J. Erythropoietin: physico- and biochemical analysis. J Chromatogr B Biomed Appl. 1996;687(1):189–199.
6. Wide L, Bengtsson C, Berglund B, Ekblom B. Detection in blood and urine of recombinant erythropoietin administered to healthy men. Med Sci Sports Exerc. 1995;27(11):1569–1576.

7. Lasne F, de Ceaurriz J. Recombinant erythropoietin in urine. Nature. 2000;405(6787):635.
8. Lasne F, Martin L, Crepin N, de Ceaurriz J. Detection of isoelectric profiles of erythropoietin in urine: differentiation of natural and administered recombinant hormones. Anal Biochem. 2002;311(2):119–126.
9. Lasne F. Double-blotting: a solution to the problem of nonspecific binding of secondary antibodies in immunoblotting procedures. J Immunol Methods. 2003;276(1–2):223–226.
10. Wide L, Bengtsson C. Molecular charge heterogeneity of human serum erythropoietin. Br J Haematol. 1990;76(1):121–127.
11. Catlin DH, Breidbach A, Elliott S, Glaspy J. Comparison of the isoelectric focusing patterns of darbepoetin alfa, recombinant human erythropoietin, and endogenous erythropoietin from human urine. Clin Chem. 2002;48(11):2057–2059.
12. Breidbach A, Catlin DH, Green GA, Tregub I, Truong H, Gorzek J. Detection of recombinant human erythropoietin in urine by isoelectric focusing. Clin Chem. 2003;49(6 Pt 1):901–907.
13. WADA technical document TD2007EPO. 2007.
14. Lasne F, Martin L, Martin JA, de CJ. Isoelectric profiles of human erythropoietin are different in serum and urine. Int J Biol Macromol. 2007;41(3):354–357.
15. Lönnberg M, Drevin M, Carlsson J. Ultra-sensitive immunochromatographic assay for quantitative determination of erythropoietin. J Immunol Methods. 2008;339(2):236–244.
16. Franke WW, Heid H. Pitfalls, errors and risks of false-positive results in urinary EPO drug tests. Clin Chim Acta. 2006;373(1–2):189–190.
17. Kahn A, Baker M. Non-specific binding of monoclonal human erythropoietin antibody AE7A5 to Escherichia coli and Saccharomyces cerevisiae proteins. Clin Chim Acta. 2006;379:173–175.
18. Beullens M, Delanghe JR, Bollen M. False-positive detection of recombinant human erythropoietin in urine following strenuous physical exercise. Blood. 2006;107(12):4711–4713.
19. Khan A, Grinyer J, Truong ST, Breen EJ, Packer NH. New urinary EPO drug testing method using two-dimensional gel electrophoresis. Clin Chim Acta. 2005;358(1–2):119–130.
20. Rabin OP, Lasne F, Pascual JA, Saugy M, Delbeke FJ, Van EP. New urinary EPO drug testing method using two-dimensional gel electrophoresis. Clin Chim Acta. 2006;373(1–2):186–187.
21. Reichel C. Identification of zinc-alpha-2-glycoprotein binding to clone AE7A5 antihuman EPO antibody by means of nano-HPLC and high-resolution high-mass accuracy ESI-MS/MS. J Mass Spectrom. 2008;43(7):916–923.
22. Peltre G, Thormann W. Evaluation Report of the Urine EPO Test. Bern: Council of the World Anti-Doping Agency (WADA); 2003.
23. Lamon S, Robinson N, Sottas PE, et al. Possible origins of undetectable EPO in urine samples. Clin Chim Acta. 2007;385(1–2):61–66.
24. Macdougall IC, Ashenden M. Current and upcoming erythropoiesis-stimulating agents, iron products, and other novel anemia medications. Adv Chronic Kidney Dis. 2009;16(2):117–130.
25. Barbone FP, Johnson DL, Farrell FX, et al. New epoetin molecules and novel therapeutic approaches. Nephrol Dial Transplant. 1999;14(Suppl 2):80–84.
26. Lamon S, Robinson N, Mangin P, Saugy M. Detection window of Darbepoetin-alpha following one single subcutaneous injection. Clin Chim Acta. 2007;379(1–2):145–149.
27. Macdougall IC. CERA (continuous erythropoietin receptor activator): a new erythropoiesis-stimulating agent for the treatment of anemia. Curr Hematol Rep. 2005;4(6):436–440.
28. Wattendorf U, Merkle HP. PEGylation as a tool for the biomedical engineering of surface modified microparticles. J Pharm Sci. 2008;97(11):4655–4669.
29. Macdougall IC. Recent advances in erythropoietic agents in renal anemia. Semin Nephrol. 2006;26(4):313–318.
30. Ashenden M, Varlet-Marie E, Lasne F, Audran M. The effects of microdose recombinant human erythropoietin regimens in athletes. Haematologica. 2006;91(8):1143–1144.
31. Caldini A, Moneti G, Fanelli A, et al. Epoetin alpha, epoetin beta and darbepoetin alfa: two-dimensional gel electrophoresis isoforms characterization and mass spectrometry analysis. Proteomics. 2003;3(6):937–941.

32. Kohler M, Ayotte C, Desharnais P, et al. Discrimination of recombinant and endogenous urinary erythropoietin by calculating relative mobility values from SDS gels. Int J Sports Med. 2008;29(1):1–6.
33. Reichel C, Kulovics R, Jordan V, Watzinger M, Geisendorfer T. SDS-PAGE of recombinant and endogenous erythropoietins: benefits and limitations of the method for application in doping control. Drug Test Anal. 2009;1:43–50.
34. Stubiger G, Marchetti M, Nagano M, Reichel C, Gmeiner G, Allmaier G. Characterisation of intact recombinant human erythropoietins applied in doping by means of planar gel electrophoretic techniques and matrix-assisted laser desorption/ionisation linear time-of-flight mass spectrometry. Rapid Commun Mass Spectrom. 2005;19(5):728–742.
35. Guan F, Uboh CE, Soma LR, et al. Differentiation and identification of recombinant human erythropoietin and darbepoetin Alfa in equine plasma by LC-MS/MS for doping control. Anal Chem. 2008;80(10):3811–3817.
36. Guan F, Uboh CE, Soma LR, Birksz E, Chen J. Identification of darbepoetin alfa in human plasma by liquid chromatography coupled to mass spectrometry for doping control. Int J Sports Med. 2009;30(2):80–86.
37. Groleau PE, Desharnais P, Cote L, Ayotte C. Low LC-MS/MS detection of glycopeptides released from pmol levels of recombinant erythropoietin using nanoflow HPLC-chip electrospray ionization. J Mass Spectrom. 2008;43(7):924–935.

Index